Stories of Hope & Healing

**Six Women
Confront
Breast
Cancer**

Stories of Hope & Healing

Six Women Confront Breast Cancer

Leslie Strong, M.D.
BREAST HEALTH PROGRAM
OF NEW YORK

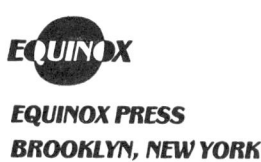

**EQUINOX PRESS
BROOKLYN, NEW YORK**

Author's Note

The names of the six principal female patients in this book, as well as the doctors and employees of the Breast Health Program, are real. All other names are fictitious, however, and no resemblance to persons living or dead is intended.

STORIES OF HOPE & HEALING: SIX WOMEN CONFRONT BREAST CANCER. Copyright © 1994 by Equinox Press. Previously published by St. Martin's Press as A Real Choice, based on the cases of Leslie Strong, M.D., © 1984 by Ralph W. Moss. Printed in the United States of America. No part of this book may be used or reproduced in any manner whatsoever without written permission except in the case of brief quotations embodied in critical articles or reviews. For information, address Equinox Press, 144 St. John's Place, Brooklyn, New York 11217, or call 718-636-1679.

Library of Congress Cataloging in Publication Data
Strong, Leslie E., M.D.
    Stories of Hope & Healing.
    1. Breast—Cancer—Psychological aspects.
2. Women—Psychology.
RC280.B8M6   1994   362.189699449   84-13268
ISBN 1-881025-07-1

First Equinox Edition
10 9 8 7 6 5 4 3 2 1

To the Women of the Breast Health Program of New York
In Gratitude and Admiration

PART ONE
Winter

Robin

New York City can be nasty in winter, with short days of sunless dreariness and moments when it might be better not to be alive. And then, suddenly, a day arrives when everyone looks around, sniffs the air, and pushes open the dusty windows, saying, "I think spring will come." You pray the weather holds and that a few feet of snow aren't waiting offshore somewhere, ready to drop on you. But while the sun shines you feel glorious—you've made it through another winter, survived, and a new year is about to blossom all around you.

It was that kind of day that found Robin Mack speeding recklessly uptown on her ten-speed bicycle. She reveled in the coolness of the breeze that whipped right through her nylon jacket and pushed her pageboy haircut back from her face. She sped through the intersection of Park and 34th, narrowly avoiding instant death at every turn. A female taxi driver honked angrily, and Robin laughed and kept on riding. She zigzagged over to the far eastern side of the island and then melted into the traffic and floated up First Avenue effortlessly.

At 65th Street she stopped at her favorite liquor store, locked the bike and deftly unsnapped the front wheel, carrying it into the store with her. Her face was cheerfulness itself, brightening the day of the two salesmen who were chatting back in the Burgundies.

"How you doin', Tony? Hey, what's a good champagne?"

Tony laughed and said something about a matter of taste and opinion. "For dinner or celebration?"

"For a celebration, a big, big celebration," she said exuberantly. She felt like pouring out the whole story for them, right there. "Something cold and something good."

She left the store with a chilled bottle of Moët, stuck it carefully in her bike pouch, and then kicked off again. She was back in the flow now, keeping up effortlessly with the cars, weaving in, through, and around them, past hospitals, flower stores, banks, antiques, and boutiques. Within twenty-five minutes of her departure from Gramercy Park she was coming up the service elevator of her building at First Avenue and 81st Street.

The door opened as soon as she rang.

"Ta da!" she cried, the champagne outstretched.

Janice, her roommate, and Peter, her boyfriend, were waiting, worried.

"What? What? What?" yelled Janice.

"Benign," Robin screamed back at her. "A cyst. Nothing!" They hugged and jumped around, and she gave Peter a long kiss.

"Dinner at The Palm," said Peter, and she was going to say no, we can't afford it, but what the hell. You only live once. And it was a glorious day, and wonderful to be alive. She loved life, and she didn't have cancer.

"Do you want to talk about it?" asked Janice. They were waiting for their rare steaks, nibbling on some wonderful home-fried potatoes Peter had ordered.

"Peter, do you mind listening to this girl talk?" Robin asked, laughing. She had a wonderful laugh, deep, throaty, intriguing. A laugh that at a certain point became indistinguishable from a sob.

Peter shrugged. He was squeamish, but couldn't admit that to her. "Sure. I'm just glad it's over and everything's okay. I told you it would be okay."

"Well, first of all, apparently it's not as hard and immobile as I thought it was. As I told you, it's a cyst. It's fairly common, a lot of women have them."

"So what does your gynecologist intend to do? Did he aspirate it?" asked Janice.

Peter bit his lip. The thought of a needle going into a woman's breast bothered him more than it seemed to bother either of the women.

"Not necessary, for now."

"Well, did he take mammograms or send you to a radiologist?"

"Listen to you," Robin said, a bit nervously. Some months back Janice had worked for a breast surgeon named Leslie Elliott Strong, helping him administer his fledgling Breast Health Program. She had become an Instant Expert on this topic. Robin was glad when that job came to an end and her roommate was on to something else.

"So what does he intend to do?"

"All he wants to do is watch it," Robin said happily. "Can you imagine? When I go back for my regular appointment in six months he'll take another look. It'll probably just disappear by itself, but if it doesn't, then he'll do something about it."

"Boy, that's a relief," said Peter.

"You said it," Robin said, laughing nervously. The steaks came—just the way they ordered them. "And don't think I wasn't worried."

She knew she had reasons to be worried. The first was her mother. Robin was a person whose life, personality, and fate seemed to parallel her mother's to an extraordinary degree. Perhaps that was why they had fought so bitterly when Robin was growing up. But they were like two peas in a pod. Robin felt an almost mystical unity with her. They had the same sense of humor. They went through life laughing. Even sorrowful things, and there were plenty, seemed to bring forth not tears but laughter, sometimes punctuated by "Please, God, help me!" or "I'm so *ill!*"

Her mother had been a singer, a dancer, and a master of ceremonies in nightclubs. Robin too had been a singer all her life—mostly jazz, soul, rhythm and blues. Then, in her twenties, she became a dancer. And now, at thirty-two, she had begun to emcee in a small club called Court Street on the Upper East Side. She ran a talent showcase, just like her mother had done. It was freaky.

They both liked to do things in a big way, a showy way, to make a splash, to spend more money than they had, to let the world know they were there. She was childish, generous, a real sucker, especially when it came to men. She had been seeing Peter for five years, longer than she had ever seen anyone. He was married—separated from a wife who refused to give him a divorce.

In 1964, just as her breasts were budding, her mother became mysteriously ill. People whispered "breast cancer." Her mother had to go in for an operation—a radical mastectomy. She seemed all right after that, but for the next fourteen years cancer was a dreaded, unspoken presence in their house in Boston. Then, in 1978, her mother was admitted to the hospital for back pains. It turned out to be cancer, the same breast cancer now widely disseminated throughout her body.

Robin rushed up to see her and walked in on her smoking. Angrily, she took the cigarettes away from her mother. Toward the end she asked her mother, "Ma, what would make you happy?"

"A cigarette," her mother whispered, and so Robin gave her one of her own.

"Take it away, it's horrible," her mother said after one drag.

It was at that point that Robin knew her mother was going to die. And in fact she did, five days later.

People whose mothers have had breast cancer are at a greater risk themselves of developing the disease, Janice had told her during her "cancerphobia" days. Their risk, in fact, was three times that of the general population of women. There were other factors going against Robin at the time she went to see her gynecologist. She was over thirty. After thirty, breast cancer becomes one of the three leading causes of death in American women (eventually rising to the number-one position in the years between forty and fifty). She lived in an urban, polluted environment. She ate rich foods and tried, at least, to maintain an affluent life-style. She smoked, although in recent years she had been cutting down.

Her gynecologist hadn't asked her about any of this, or warned her about any risks. She only knew it because of her crazy roommate and her old boss, Dr. Strong. But the important thing was that he *had* examined her, and everything was okay. As long as it wasn't malignant.

Dr. Strong

Dr. Strong leaned back in his Brooklyn office and closed his eyes. It had been one of those frenetic days. He had operated on two patients at Beth Israel that morning, then run out to Forest Hills to discuss the Breast Health Program with a group of executives. Then back to Brooklyn on the BQE just in time for his afternoon appointments. It was a rainy Tuesday, and the drizzle came down insistently over the city, painting everything gray, like a muddied watercolor. He could hear the hiss of rush-hour traffic outside his window on Prospect Park West. A shred of daylight hung tenaciously over the park.

He had to return a few calls from doctors—"feeders" who referred cases to him. That would be it. He'd rush home to East End Avenue, shower, and then have a leisurely dinner with his friend Dorothy Wayner at a little hole-in-the-wall on Third Avenue with delicious Czech-German food. He looked forward to a few hours of peace, of warmth, and a good night's sleep.

Suddenly, the outside doorbell rang. He opened his eyes and became aware of a car parked at the curb, its amber lights flashing. It could be a patient of the internist with whom he shared the suite. But a moment later his interoffice buzzer rang and his receptionist/nurse, Susan Fisherman, said,

"There's a Ms. Jill Highland* here to see you, Dr. Strong."

Strong checked his jam-packed notebook nervously. Had he forgotten a last appointment? But no, he had definitely seen his final scheduled appointment for the day.

"Are you sure it's for me?"

"Ms. Jill Highland," said the receptionist.

"Well, make an appointment for next Tuesday. I'm done for the day. Literally."

There was a long pause. "She says it's an emergency," said the receptionist. There was an unaccustomed edge to her voice, probably a reflection of the patient's own nervousness. This was strange, a bit intriguing. There weren't many "emergencies" in Strong's line of medicine. The "emergency" was usually just a sudden panic attack upon discovering a lump.

"All right, show her in."

A moment later a woman entered, with a man in tow. Both of them were young, well-dressed, probably wealthy. The woman was a fine-looking blonde and wore an expensive fur coat.

"Thank you for seeing me," said the woman, making a determined effort to be charming. "My name is Jill Highland. I'm sorry to come with no prior appointment. But it was an emergency."

Strong nodded noncommitally.

"I got your name from Dr. Farrell,* my gynecologist." Strong was interested. Farrell had never sent him a patient before, but this could be a good lead, as Brandt Farrell had a large, established, and prosperous practice in Brooklyn.

"And what's the emergency?"

"Well, I'm going away, to the islands, this weekend, and Dr. Farrell just insisted that I see someone about this infection. I would like it taken care of before I go."

It sounded a bit like she was ordering something from the caterers.

"An infection?" asked Strong. Breast infections were not uncommon, but why would an experienced man like Farrell send a patient to him? And why such urgency? "Have you taken anything for it?"

*Name changed.

"Of course. Dr. Farrell has given me two antibiotics, but neither has done any good. It's really becoming a bit bothersome." She glanced nervously over at her companion, who took her hand.

"Are you married?" Strong asked suddenly.

"What? Oh, I'm sorry. How gauche of me! This is my fiancé, Grant Mellor."

"Well, if you don't mind, Mr. Mellor, you can stay here while I examine your fiancée. Let's have a look at you."

He led the way down the long corridor.

"Both breasts?" Strong asked.

"No, it's just this one—the right one." Strong stared. Even before she disrobed he thought that he could see through the blouse and detect something . . . well, peculiar, not right.

Already he was worried. "When did you get this infection?"

"When could it have been? About two months ago. Nine weeks, to be exact."

He closed the door. "Okay, let's have a look at it. You can put your blouse and bra on that chair, if you don't mind." She glanced nervously at the anatomical drawings on the wall, the ones he used to illustrate breast illnesses to his patients.

"Do you want me to remove it all?" she asked. He nodded and occupied himself arranging instruments on a tray—busy work. When he turned around he knew, in an instant, that this beautiful woman's life was in serious jeopardy. He couldn't be absolutely positive, but he had seen it a number of times before, and the diagnosis just screamed out at him: inflammatory CA.

He winced, but quickly recovered. He would have to be clear and accurate.

Inflammatory cancer was first described in the early 1800s, he recalled. Although it constituted only about three percent of breast surgeons' practice, it was something they all particularly dreaded. For other kinds of breast disease, including carcinoma, there were odds, treatments, variables. Inflammatory CA, on the other hand, was implacable. The textbook said, emotionlessly, that "the duration of symptoms averaged four to six months." What a delicate way of saying this young woman would almost certainly be dead before the leaves fell from the trees.

That is if his diagnosis, which was little more than a gut reaction, was really correct. In cases like this he prayed that his appraisal was incorrect—which was something like a jockey betting against his own horse. He examined her more closely. It was a classical case all right. The skin over the affected breast was swollen and fiery red. It had begun to take on what doctors called a *peau d'orange* texture—"orange peel" in French. To heighten the pathos, the other breast was simply beautiful. It had a natural swoop, a lovely untouched nipple. The affected breast was hard and practically frozen to the chest wall. When he had Jill lie down on the examining table, it stood up, unyielding.

Nice of Dr. Farrell to wait all these weeks before sending her over, Strong thought angrily.

Well, he would do a biopsy to make sure. Cancer in the small lymphatic vessels of the skin would clinch it. Maybe he was wrong. But all his instincts and training told him she had it.

He said nothing, but walked with her silently back to the office. He tried to compose a speech. These were the moments he most dreaded about being a doctor. He wouldn't deny that he loved the life of a surgeon. Yes, it was a power trip, but he had the power to help people, to save them, to earn their gratitude. Being a doctor satisfied needs that were deeply embedded in him. Yet here he was, an expert on breast cancer, and he was totally helpless to affect the course of this woman's illness. He might as well have been a primitive medicine man! He felt a terrible, unfocused anger at those dark, unknown, unseen forces that so blithely struck down these women in their prime.

How was he going to tell her? What words could he find? Some doctors simply ran away from the problem, refusing to deal with it. Others became stone-cold and clinical, refusing to show any human emotion. Or they wrapped themselves in a cynical veneer. None of these reactions were very satisfactory, especially for the patient. Strong did not want to yield his humanity to this monster disease, yet it exacted an enormous toll from him.

"Listen, I have some disturbing news for you," Strong began. "I don't think this is a simple infection. It's been with you for over two months and it hasn't responded yet to antibiotics. I think we need to do some further tests."

The woman sat on the edge of her chair. "What sort of tests?"

"Well, I'd like to admit you to a hospital and do some procedures. Primarily, Jill, I'd like you to have a biopsy of that skin."

"A biopsy sounds like cancer," she said.

"It's a possibility," said Strong, trying not to look away as he said it.

"I think you must be mistaken, Dr. Strong," said her fiancé, agitated now. His mature and rational pose was quickly evaporating. He was a kid in a three-piece suit.

"It's a very minor operation, really," said Strong, trying to sound reassuring. "All I'll do is take a small piece of skin."

"This is ridiculous," said Jill, her voice breaking nervously. "Come on, let's get out of here."

"Listen to me," said Strong, exasperated. "This is extremely serious. I'm afraid you may have a very dangerous form of malignancy. It's imperative that you get a biopsy taken immediately."

"I think there's far too much surgery in the world already. Far too many surgeons and far too much surgery," said Jill angrily.

"Perhaps," said Strong. "But that doesn't change the facts in your case." He decided to try a different tack. "I'll tell you what. Instead of going in for surgery, tomorrow go for a second opinion. I'll give you the names of three or four other surgeons. If they agree, will you go in for a biopsy?"

It was a gamble—she might just hit on someone who failed to recognize the symptoms—but what else could he do?

"This is ridiculous," she said finally. She stood up to go. Her fiancé looked at Strong with a mixture of defiance and apology. Strong could imagine how he felt, the conflicts.

"I'll find a doctor who'll treat me for my infection," she said. "All of this is silly."

He had just a moment now to try and save her. There were new therapies all the time, he argued, new ideas, new treatments. "Just sit down, Jill. What does it take to convince you?" Despair was creeping into his voice. "I'll do whatever you want. Just don't walk away from it."

But it was too late. She swept out of the office without a

backward look. Strong stood at the window and watched their car pull away from the curb, its red stop lights now making garish neon streaks on the avenue. Soon it was gone, just another car in the stream of traffic. People on their way home to warmth, safety, and security. The sky over Prospect Park had lost even a hint of iridescence. Night came early in January.

Yes, he would get into his Buick Regal and fight his own way through Flatbush Avenue traffic, over the Manhattan Bridge. With luck he would be home in under an hour. Then a quiet dinner with Dorothy.

He pushed his chair back, emotionally drained, and leaned his head back on the padded chair. The sounds of the office and the street sounded far away. He could smell the desk. Some things in life were very puzzling. He didn't know how long he sat like that, but when he lifted his head he was surprised to find that his cheeks were wet with tears.

It was because of women like Jill—frightened, confused, ill-informed—that he had started the Breast Health Program of New York a year before. He remembered clearly how it had begun. One Saturday morning he awoke early—it was a habit he couldn't break even on weekends—and took the crosstown bus to the Claremont Stables. Claremont, near Central Park West, was the last stable left in Manhattan. For a reasonable fee, he could take a horse out for an hour or so. It was early in the year, but the weather was crisp and clean, and when he mounted Suntan he even felt a trifle warm in his cable-knit sweater and plaid jacket. He needed to get away from everything to think.

Strong had been riding Suntan for years. He was a high-spirited horse, but, if you respected his feelings, very good and responsive. He loved the feeling of being in communion with this powerful being, the press of his silky sides against his legs, the incredible energy. He could never understand how his Buick could have over 300 *horse*power. One horse, such as Suntan, seemed so much more powerful than any car.

The grooms backed away as they went through the wooden stable gate: Suntan had a "bad rep" and had thrown more than one of them. Strong smiled, both a friendly smile and a smile of amusement. He didn't have any trouble with this animal. He respected its independence, and he hoped the feeling was mutual.

They clip-clopped out onto the bridle path and sauntered along for a while. The morning sun filtered through the last remaining leaves. This was a time to relax, but, in fact, it was very difficult for Leslie Strong ever really to relax. His ex-wife called him a workaholic. Sometimes he believed that overwork had given him his prematurely gray and thinning hair. In fact, his son had once asked him if he had lost his hair by pulling it out in aggravation. He had laughed—such things were genetically determined, of course, but he couldn't help feeling that his way of life had aged him more than it had many of his contemporaries. Breast surgery was, as they said, a hell of a way to make a living, especially if you became emotionally involved with your patients, as he invariably did.

Strong was particularly troubled this morning. He nudged the horse onto the shaded path and gave a shake of the reins. Suntan picked up speed effortlessly. Strong knew what the focus of his concern was: there seemed to be something wrong with his practice of medicine. Not that he wasn't doing his best. As a surgeon he knew he was good. He saw the work of other doctors and never felt at a loss. He counseled women well, and they seemed to like him. But something was missing.

He thought about all the women he had seen who were so terrified of the whole topic of breast disease that they fled the doctor. Other more "rational" women reacted in similar ways: by delaying treatment, making wrong decisions, all because of ignorance and fear.

But it's not just the women, he thought. There was also a problem with the doctors. He thought about a case he had had recently—Ernestine Merryman. He summoned up an image of her in his mind: her cherubic, somewhat overweight black face. A really lovely person, but terribly uneducated about her body and particularly her breasts. What a story she had told!

She came clutching a note on the stationery of her gynecologist, a man who had sent him a few patients before. The note said simply that "Ernestine Merryman has been under my care for suspicion of carcinoma." Just like that. Strong had studied the note, a bit incredulously. He noticed immediately that Ernestine hadn't brought anyone to the office with her. He was very sensitive to these unconscious signals and this was almost always a bad sign. A lack of concerned relatives made the whole process more difficult for both the patient and the doctor. He always liked to have relatives or close friends as a backup.

"Are you all alone in New York?" he had asked.

"No," she answered slowly, in the cadence of the South. "I live with my mother in the Bronx. But I see no reason to get her involved in this."

When Strong examined her, he got another shock. The woman removed her ample brassiere, and he was amazed to see that she had already been operated on, the crude black sutures still in place.

"What is this?" he asked, almost shrieked, he was so surprised.

Ernestine began to sob. "I don't know. . . . The doctor did this to me."

"The gynecologist *did* this?" Strong asked, examining the cut. "He did the biopsy? When? Where?"

"He told me he could do the operation himself," she said, daubing her eyes with a tissue. "In his office. But now he tells me I have to get a surgeon. They told me at the clinic you were a breast doctor."

Strong stared at this woman incredulously. Then he felt a sudden surge of rage. The idea of gynecologists doing breast surgery—even biopsies—was outrageous to him.

"I don't do pelvic examinations," he said angrily. "Where does he come off doing breast surgery? Don't you realize he's not qualified? Didn't you question this? Why didn't you go immediately to a breast specialist?"

He couldn't help himself: he was yelling at this poor woman, yet of course it wasn't her fault. She listened to the doctor, because doctor knows best.

"Didn't he give you anything else to bring with you?" asked Strong.

"Yes, he gave me this chart." She fished into her large imitation-leather bag and came up with a pathology report from a local laboratory. It said, "Analysis of specimen: Infiltrating Medullary Carcinoma of the Breast."

"My God," said Strong. The implications of this case were

staggering. First of all, the specimen was undoubtedly gone. It had been done by a laboratory of questionable accuracy, and the correctness of the diagnosis was not at all certain. Second, the gynecologist had fouled up his operating field. He had possibly removed some nodes or lymph glands, as well, in the process. If these nodes had been positive, then the patient would need chemotherapy. But if he happened to remove the only positive nodes, then no one would ever know of this regional involvement, and she wouldn't get chemotherapy. In a young woman with nodal involvement, chemotherapy could add years to her survival time. The chemotherapist would have his hands full with this one.

Also, reconstruction would now become much more difficult because of the mess this OB-GYN had left behind. And in a big-busted woman like this, reconstruction would become very important. People would definitely notice the absence of one breast.

Strong examined the wound and felt the nodes. There seemed to be regional involvement already. This was going to be hard: he wished the woman's mother or some other relative was with her. Dealing with women who presented themselves totally alone was usually difficult—and very, very sad.

"Ernestine, did the gynecologist tell you what this means?" he asked, holding up the piece of notepaper that served as her calling card.

She shook her head. "He just said I should see another doctor, a surgeon."

"Do you know you have cancer?"

She shook her head slowly. "Does that mean I'm going to die?" Her large eyes reflected her fear.

"No, it doesn't," said Strong, trying to sound as positive as he could. "But you're going to need further surgery. We're going to have to remove your breast. It's called a mastectomy."

Ernestine caught her pointer finger between her teeth and bit down hard. Strong thought she was going to draw blood.

"Do whatever you have to do, doctor," she said, her eyes averted.

Well, at least he would have a chance at saving her. But how sick he was of hearing that! He didn't want to play God, although he knew that that was why some people became doctors in the first place. But how could he educate these women who often behave like passive lumps of clay in the hands of various physicians? That was the question.

His concern for Ernestine Merryman as an individual had begun to merge with general questions about his practice of surgery. Breast cancer was such a complicated disease and so many new treatment alternatives were opening up all the time that it required a great deal of intelligence and knowledge on the part of both the doctor and the patient to reach an informed decision. He realized that, but how could he help the women to understand that? Most of them were still ignorant about the question of breast disease, or, because they were fearful, had an ostrichlike attitude toward the problem.

His horse quickened its pace and came up alongside another Claremont horse, a female. They were on the stretch of track that adjoined the Brambles. On the other horse, which Strong recognized from its dark black color as Manchego, was a woman in her mid-thirties.

"Beautiful morning, isn't it?" asked Strong.

She turned around, a bit startled. She, too, was alone and apparently, like him, used this time to go deep into her private thoughts.

"For this time of year it certainly is," she said, regaining her composure.

Strong could tell she was an experienced rider. English saddle is not easy, and she handled the horse with a degree of mastery he immediately admired. Suntan fell behind, and Strong spurred him on to catch up again.

"Come here often?" he asked, drawing up beside her. It had not escaped his notice that this particular woman was also very good-looking. He had little time to socialize or meet women, and he wasn't about to let this opportunity pass. In fact, in the back of his mind, these morning horseback rides always figured as a possible way of meeting new people. So far, however, he hadn't had much success. New York, contrary to popular opinion, is not always kind to unattached people.

"Every week," she said. "I usually don't come this early, though."

"No," said Strong, "or else I probably would have met you before. I'm sure I would have noticed you, too."

She smiled. "My name's Dorothy Wayner," she said, reaching over her hand. Shaking under such conditions was comical —they were both in imminent danger of becoming unsaddled— and they laughed.

"Leslie Strong," he said.

"Do you live in the city?" he asked.

"Yes, I do," she said. "I work in midtown and live on the East Side. It's nice. I can walk to work if the weather's nice."

"That's great," said Strong, not knowing exactly what to say, but afraid to say nothing. He didn't want to lose her so quickly. "What do you do?"

"I'm basically in public relations," she said. "And also advertising. I'm a vice-president of Sawdon and Bess. And you?"

"I'm a breast surgeon," said Strong.

"At what hospital?" she asked, a bit surprised. Perhaps he didn't live up to her image of breast surgeons, he thought.

"I'm in private practice," he said. "But I have admitting privileges at Beth Israel and Mount Sinai, as well as Methodist in Brooklyn."

"Do you like your work?" she asked after a pause. He was glad she asked it, too, because not only did he like to talk about it, but it showed that she was interested in him.

"Well, I wonder every morning when I wake up," he said. "I used to be a professor of surgery. Going into private practice was quite a change. But actually I love surgery. It may sound corny, but I like helping people. But it's also got its bad points."

"I can imagine," she said emphatically.

"It's not what you think," said Strong. "Not just seeing so much pain, but, well, I was just this minute thinking about this question—the ignorance of so many women, as well as their doctors, especially their gynecologists on this whole question of treating breast disease. It's become quite complicated in the last few years, but people's thinking and attitudes have not generally kept up."

They rode along, and Leslie Strong explained to Dorothy about the problems he had been encountering. When they got to the stable, the horses tried to enter, but they reined them to the left and back onto the path. They had agreed—almost without words—to go around for another hour.

"Are you the only one who feels like this?" she asked.

"Are you kidding? I know a dozen other doctors—surgeons, radiologists, oncologists—who are also disgusted with the lack of understanding. Not that things can't be done for women with breast disease. On the contrary, new modalities are coming into existence all the time. Alternatives. For instance, I'm sure you've heard it's no longer necessary to do a radical mastectomy on all patients, as they did in the old days. It's been quite a revolution in the last ten years. Nowadays, you do a modified radical in almost all cases, or a quadrant resection, or even a lumpectomy."

Dorothy laughed. "Whoa," she said, "slow down." (Manchego, ever attentive, turned her ears around at this.) "I'm not familiar with these terms. But I get the overall picture: medicine is making progress, but the news of that progress hasn't gotten out to the public yet."

"Exactly," Strong almost shouted. "I love the way you put things, Dorothy." From someone else it would have sounded phony—like a come-on. But Strong's nature was basically very enthusiastic and almost naive. He especially appreciated other people's fine points. And he held people with an easy command of language almost in awe.

"But what's wrong with going to a cancer center or specialized hospital?" Dorothy asked.

"Well, first of all, the patient often gets lost in the shuffle. Sometimes they don't even see the same doctor twice. They're a number, a statistic. That's bad enough at the motor-vehicle bureau," he said, laughing, "and there your life doesn't depend on it. But with breast cancer, it often does.

"Also, the cancer centers treat people, but they don't usually offer education so patients can choose the best alternative. They make all the decisions for you, and sometimes you aren't even informed of what's going on."

"I know what you're talking about," Dorothy said. "I know quite a lot about hospitals."

"Then, at the big centers, the breast surgeons sometimes neglect the other aspects of treatment. For instance, patients don't get to consult with the radiologist before the surgery, to see if their kind of problem could better be handled with radiation. There's a lot of rivalry, you know. And after the surgery they often don't send the patient to a plastic surgeon to discuss reconstruction."

"Why is that?"

"Well, a lot of guys feel that reconstruction interferes with their ability to detect recurrences. They set the patients' cosmetic appearance at next to nothing. To me it's very important. This case I was telling you about—the young black woman—I'm sending her to see a plastic surgeon right away, so that I can adjust my surgery according to what he feels can be done afterward."

"That's very good," said Dorothy. She dismounted and walked the horse for a bit. They had been out for almost two hours. As she got off Strong was shocked: she walked with a pronounced limp in one leg, in fact, it seemed almost immobile. "Oh," she said, casually noticing his stare. "I had polio when I was ten," she said.

"That's amazing," he said, a bit embarrassed at having stared. "Well, then, how—how did you ever learn to ride like you do? I mean, I never would have known."

She laughed. "I learned to ride before I got polio, as a kid growing up on Long Island. And then, afterward, I went back to it as therapy. I've gotten pretty good at it, I think."

"I should say," said Leslie. He swung off Suntan and walked alongside her. "That's terrific."

"I also ice skate," she said, trying to sound modest, but glowing with her pride.

"I bet you're good at that, too," he said.

"Not bad. The next question is how I manage it, right? Well, I just skate along on the bad leg and guide myself with the good. It's really simpler than it sounds."

He stared at her in admiration. "So you're a person who knows something about medicine."

"And about the problems patients face," she said. "You know, I would like to help you if I can," she said decisively.

"That would be wonderful. What do you have in mind?"

"Well, I've had some experience in publicizing public interest groups. I've also been involved with women's health organizations. I think what you're saying all boils down to one thing: public education. You want to educate women, other doctors, and the general public about what needs to be done."

"For breast disease," he said, nodding vigorously.

"For breast *health*," she corrected him. "You need a preventive approach, a positive approach. Listen, Leslie, why don't we meet and talk sometime next week."

"Perhaps we could have dinner?" They had approached the stables again, and Suntan and Manchego, this time, would brook no interference. They pulled vigorously toward the gate. "This is very exciting. I'm so happy I met you, Dorothy. I can't believe I almost didn't come here this morning! Can you imagine!"

She laughed, flattered. "I hope you won't think I'm too bold, but why do we have to wait until next week? How about this weekend? How about tonight?"

That evening, at seven o'clock, Strong was waiting by the door of her apartment. He was dressed in his Italian silk suit and had brought her a bunch of flowers he had grabbed at the last minute from a twenty-four-hour fruit-and-vegetable stand on her corner.

They talked until past midnight, about themselves, their families, their hopes and dreams. But they also talked about business, the business of educating the public about breast health. Out of this discussion the Breast Health Program of New York was born.

Christine

On a sunny winter day, at precisely noon, Christine Mackin left her brownstone house on Montgomery Street and bounded toward Prospect Park. She jogged gently along Prospect Park West, moving her arms in limbering motions. Off in the distance the Soldiers' and Sailors' monument of Grand Army Plaza seemed diaphanous, its blue-green colors breaking into brightly colored dots in the direct sunlight.

There were entrances about one hundred yards away on either side of her, but, eager to start, Chris jumped up onto one of the crumbling benches and, after testing the wood with her foot, leaped from the top rung of the bench into the park.

She walked briskly through the musty-smelling grove, glancing briefly at an old newspaper now rotting into the soil:

CARDINAL COOKE
DYING OF LEUKEMIA

An inside page had been flapped open by the wind. "The Point of Death," it screamed. She wondered what the *Post* columnists could possibly have to say about the "point of death." The whole ghoulish subject bothered her.

She went through her warm-up exercises. Ridiculous to be

morbid on such a brilliant day. Live for the present. It is the only world we've got, and we only pass this way once.

She bounded across the outer road and ran down the incline till she had an unobstructed view of the Long Meadow. Running the circumference of the park every day had given her a new appreciation of its beauty.

To her husband, John, it was an odd assortment of trees and ratty lawns. He was dubious about its clientele and wondered about the wisdom of Chris jogging there. John cared about the investment value of their brownstone, but for her, the important thing was to be near the park itself, so that she could run in it all four seasons of the year.

In the early afternoon, the park was virtually deserted. She would make the whole circuit, past the lake, the tasteless Wollman skating rink, stopping in to visit with the somewhat pathetic pachyderms at the zoo. It was seedy, of course, but its very neglect attracted her. She dreaded tasteless modernization more than benign neglect.

As she jogged, attaining her optimum speed now, she observed her fellow park lovers. Chris was a people-watcher. She hated sports in which you had no contact with the outside world, such as swimming or squash. How boring to stare at four walls, without a breath of fresh air or a glimpse of something new and interesting.

She ran up the first hill, past the benches filled with sad-looking unemployed men. John had come with her once and had been horrified at the sight of a man attempting to wash himself at one of the concrete water basins. But nobody ever bothered her here. Perhaps, with her short hair, her square jaw, and her powerful-looking legs, she was too tough-looking to entice any muggers.

As she ran, the sweat began to pour off her. She loved that feeling. If she didn't return home soaking, she didn't feel as if she had run. The big race, the local marathon, was coming up, too, and she had to be in top shape. She would finish her run in an hour, then go home for a light lunch. As she moved along, she thought of food, of blueberries and yogurt and wheat germ.

A squirrel ran across her path, then another—the male, no doubt—in hot pursuit. A lanky, expensive-looking dog fetched a stick thrown by a master who remained invisible to her behind a small rise in the terminal moraine.

The air smelled sweet with the perfume of decomposing leaves under the snow. The sky was a milky blue, fringed by swift-moving clouds.

She was halfway through the run, coming along the lake, with a startling view of the Brooklyn Museum in the distance, when she had an unpleasant sensation. She was wearing a new brassiere, supposed to be specially designed for runners, but the sweat and motion had loosened it. She would have to stop and fix it. There was no one in her immediate vicinity: the closest people were a group of teenagers lolling by the fringe of the lake.

She reached into her sweaty bra to adjust the strap and her hand froze. Inside the right cup, close to her breastbone, she felt something. She withdrew her hand and decided to try again. She reached in and touched the area. At first she felt nothing, but then, just as she was about to expel her held-in breath in relief, there it was again. A definite lump. It didn't hurt. She poked it a little bit. It was small, about the size of a chickpea, perhaps, but the sweat on her face went cold suddenly. "Where the hell did that come from?" she said—unaware that she was talking out loud.

It can't be. She started jogging again, and ran about one hundred yards before she stopped. She reached in again, but it was still there. *It's nothing, nothing at all. It'll probably go away in a couple of days.* That self-assurance didn't last, however. By the time she got within sight of Grand Army Plaza, she felt sick to her stomach and had to stop. She sat on a bench, light-headed, her head drooping between her muscular thighs. This was incredible. But look, she told herself, most of these things turn out to be perfectly harmless. Every lump and bump is not necessarily cancer. Her father, for instance, had had half a dozen bumps like this in his arms for years. They had never even been removed. Undoubtedly this was just like that.

She ran on, feeling better, but was glad when she reached the steps of her house and got inside. She locked herself in the bathroom and stripped off her soaking blouse and her bra. Her cat's paw came under the bathroom door, but she ignored it. She felt along the breastbone carefully, her fingers delineating the new growth. It wasn't so large, not even as large as it had seemed in the park.

Surely this was nothing.

Her short-lived optimism disappeared, however, when she examined the other breast, the left one. There were two other growths already poking out of that one, each of them bigger and more menacing than the first.

Christine made an appointment to see Dr. Kenneth Jaffe, her internist and family physician in Park Slope. Jaffe felt the lumps. To him they were not alarming—many women Christine's age had breast lumps, and most times they turned out to be benign. Nevertheless, they couldn't be ignored, and so he recommended that she immediately go to see Dr. Strong, whom he knew from Methodist Hospital.

John came with her to Strong's office, which was practically around the corner from their house. After the examination, Christine and John sat in the consultation room of Strong's office. Luckily, it was the night of Melanie's dance class on Seventh Avenue, and they had arranged for her to stay with the teacher if they were late.

"It's bad news, isn't it?" said Chris. "Three lumps. One of them's bound to be cancer, huh?"

"Not necessarily," said Strong. "In fact, most lumps that are discovered in breast examinations are benign. You understand 'benign'?"

"Noncancerous," said John.

"Precisely. The most common breast disease, in fact, is fibrocystic disease. This is predominantly found in women your age, Christine. The twenty-five-to-forty-five age group. It's characterized by what we call nodularity and a general thickening of breast tissue as well as a lumpiness to the breast."

"Is that what I have?"

"You *do* have that condition, yes," said Strong. "Many women do—some people say more than twenty-five percent of American women have it. The cysts that accompany this condition are benign, however, and are treated simply by needle aspiration."

Chris let out a sigh: that wasn't so bad. They stick a needle in, draw out the fluid, and it went away—almost like pricking a blister.

"Not so fast," said Strong. "I said you *had* this condition, but I didn't say that was the cause of these three lumps. Fibrocystic disease is your background condition, if you will. But let's take this step by step."

Christine squirmed. Her mind just didn't work this way. She wanted to get to the issue—did she need surgery? Did she have cancer?—and skip the fancy talk. But John was interested, in his methodical, very male way.

"What you appear to have," said Strong, "is a fibroadenoma." John wrote this down on the little note pad he had bought for the occasion. "This is another common benign breast tumor. It appears as a solid, localized, noncystic, mobile, and well-circumscribed tumor. That is what your lumps appear to be."

"So I don't have cancer?"

"Probably not," said Strong.

"Then I won't need surgery," she said.

"Not true," said Strong, in that blunt, telegraphic style he shared with many surgeons and people of action in general. "Our principle is that a biopsy should be performed on all tumors palpable on breast examination, or that are revealed only by mammograms and not on physical examination. In your case, the tumors are quite visible on physical examination, and also will undoubtedly show up on the mammograms I will have you take."

"Does that mean going into the hospital?" asked John.

"Yeah, I'd like to avoid that if I can," Christine added. She just didn't want to be away from Melanie, since she dreaded the effect that might have on her daughter.

"I'm coming to that," said Strong. "Please just listen and pay attention. There are two types of biopsies. First, an excisional biopsy. This involves the complete removal of the tumor, not just a portion of it. This is immediately submitted to a pathologist who performs a frozen section and can tell the surgeon—within minutes—the nature of the problem. On the other hand, there is also an incisional biopsy, which involves the removal of a portion of the tumor. Since it only removes a portion, a slice of the tumor, it's not as accurate, since cancer cells could still be present in the remaining portion. Is that clear?"

"I thought you said it wasn't cancer," said Christine, her normal happy expression gone.

"Back up," said Strong. Why did this always happen, he wondered. No matter how clear he made things, people continued to hear what they wanted to hear. "I said these tumors *probably* weren't cancer. The odds are in your favor."

"Thanks," said Chris, ironically.

"Greatly in your favor. But that's why we perform the biopsy, to find out for sure."

"It sounds as if the excisional biopsy is more thorough," said John.

"Most breast specialists today prefer to do the excisional biopsy," said Strong, "because of its accuracy and completeness."

"Would that mean going into the hospital? I have an eleven-year-old at home. . . ."

"Most breast biopsies can be performed under local anesthesia, or general anesthesia, even on an ambulatory outpatient basis," said Strong. "But for many reasons I still prefer to have you stay in the hospital for a day or two. That way you can get your mammograms done the night before, and can rest up afterward. I mean, it is minor surgery, but it's still surgery, and it's more convenient for me and any other doctors to come to you than for you to have to come to us."

"Don't worry," said John, directing himself to Chris, "I'll watch after Melanie. She'll be fine. Better to have it done right, if you're going to have it done at all."

"Why is there such an emphasis on mammograms?" asked Christine. "There seems to be so much confusion about them nowadays."

"Well, there has been a lot of confusion, that's true. But mammography is the only technique we have at the present time that can detect a breast tumor and the characteristics of the tumor—to help tell if it's benign or malignant. A breast self-examination can often find a lump, as you discovered yours, but it rarely reveals whether it's cancer or not. But a mammogram does other things. Basically, the mammogram adds a tremendous amount of information to a breast examination. In my opinion, which is also the opinion of the American Cancer Society, *all* women thirty-five years old or older should have a mammogram and repeat it every five years on a routine basis up to the age of fifty."

"Hold it," said John. "What do you need a mammogram for if you're already doing the biopsy?"

"Good point," said Strong. "The mammogram they do in the hospital is not primarily done for the breast that the tumor is in, but to provide information about the *opposite* breast. You see, very often the breasts are like mirror images of each other, and a problem that develops in one breast has its corresponding problem in the other breast. We want to know if that's the case before we operate. In your wife's case, we already know that there is a problem in both breasts, but we want to find out the extent of the problem."

"But isn't mammography dangerous?" asked Christine. "I read an article about that once."

"Well, in my opinion mammography does not increase one's risk of developing breast cancer. The amount of radiation involved is minute, and is about one-tenth of what it was ten years ago. The average mammogram today, with ultrasensitive films, involves less than half a rad of radiation."

"Is the biopsy a big operation?" she asked nervously.

"Not at all," said Strong. "It's really rather minor. I'll be very careful with the stitches, so that in a year or so you'll hardly know you were operated on."

"I don't know. . . ." she said, hesitating.

"You're making more out of this than there is. We'll put a few little bandages on it and we'll have you back to your routine in no time," said Strong. The important thing was to get her into the hospital, he felt.

"All right," said Christine finally. "I guess it will be all right. I just have so many bad associations with hospitals. My mother died when I was very young—when she was young, too."

"She did?" asked Strong, a bit apprehensive. "What did she die of?"

Chris bit her lip. It had happened so many years ago, yet it remained so vivid. "I don't really know," she said. "I'm not lying, but, you see, I was young, and they never really told us. I know she had an operation of some kind, and there were rumors. Does it matter?"

"What kind of rumors?" asked Strong.

"Well, I remember people saying that she had . . . cancer."

Strong closed his eyes for a moment. "Breast cancer?"

"I don't know," said Christine.

"You don't know what your mother died of?" Strong asked, incredulous.

"I was very young, Dr. Strong," she said. "Is it important?"

"It could be," said Strong. "It could affect your prognosis and maybe even your treatment."

Chris swallowed hard. "Well, if it's important, I guess I could find out."

She had come this way many times before. Often she would jog past Methodist Hospital, but since the construction of the new wing, on Eighth Avenue, she had found other routes: the noise and dust had made this part of the street unpleasant for running for a while.

Now she was here again, but this time as a patient. After parking the car in the lot around the corner, John helped her with her bags into the waiting room that adjoined the lobby. He was being incredibly understanding these days, in a way almost too much so, since his solicitousness made her suspect that her condition was even worse than she was being told.

They were early and there were a few families ahead of them waiting to check in their loved ones. Restless, Chris got up and started to meander around the lobby of the hospital, looking at the plaques on the walls, trying to gauge the history of the place or at least its self-image.

"First Methodist Hospital in America," said one.

Whoop-de-doo, she thought.

A dog barked outside—a Dachshund tied to the gate, its breath rising in white puffs. No one seemed to mind. Outside, the bright air was filled with the urban noises of Brooklyn—a muffled jackhammer, the wail of an ambulance (three of which were parked by the front entrance), the hum of a generator. They were pouring concrete to the left of the main entrance, unloading clanging window frames to the right.

Yet despite the turmoil, the air outside had smelled surprisingly sweet. How she would like to be out there, free, running through the park, her muscles pumping, feeling the sweat pouring off her body and soaking her sweatshirt. She felt a sudden impulse to flee. What the hell was she doing here, anyway? she wondered. This is crazy. There's nothing wrong with me.

"Christine Mackin," said a voice.

She turned. It was a volunteer, a silver-haired old woman with a Methodist patch on her jacket.

"They want you in admitting now, dear," she said.

John picked up her bag, and they followed the woman into the admissions office, past the Phillips Chapel, which smelled of wax, past the "wishing well" made of cardboard that had garnered a few nickels and pennies from the superstitious.

She was admitted without incident and taken up to her room. Her roommate was having a hysterectomy. Luckily, she was a pleasant and quiet woman around fifty years old, whose son was in the navy, at the moment, she informed Chris proudly, in a submarine several thousand feet under the North Atlantic. She had a picture of the boy, with his wide-open teenager face, sitting on her table, No other relatives.

Chris paid three dollars for the TV to be hooked up and then gave her wallet to the desk nurse for safekeeping. John had to get to work but said he would come by again, and by six o'clock he was there, with what must have been an outrageously expensive bouquet of flowers. He was in a playful mood, and at one point stuck his hand under the covers and made her scream. She enjoyed the attention. Somehow, with him there, the whole thing seemed so absurd. After all, she wasn't sick.

"You gotta do this," he said, putting his feet up on the edge of the bed. "But I spoke to Dr. Strong. He says in your age category the chances are it's nothing serious. In a week or two you'll forget all about it."

The next morning they shaved her and took her upstairs to the ninth floor, the surgical floor.

"Is that my patient?" someone yelled. It was Dr. Strong. "How are you feeling this morning, Christine?" he asked.

"I'm okay," she said, and she meant it.

"Good, you seem okay. We'll have you running again in no time at all, don't worry," he said jovially. She watched him go down the hall, greeting almost every person he met.

They wheeled her directly into the operating room. The anesthesiologist and his attentive resident added another line to her I.V. drip, a sedative.

"Tell me when you taste the garlic," said the anesthesiologist. "Say 'I taste the garlic.' "

She wondered what this meant. Was it some secret code? Garlic? Maybe anesthetics are made from garlic, she thought, and the idea amused her. She was starting to float.

Suddenly she did taste it. "I taste the gar—" she said. She

pushed hard to get the "—lic," but it wouldn't form on her lips. She struggled for what seemed an endless moment, and then went into a deep sleep, never having finished the word.

She dreamed about her mother.

She is back in her father's house in the Carroll Gardens section of Brooklyn.

The house is perfectly still. It is afternoon, late afternoon, and she is watching the mites of dust filtering through the warm sunlight. There is a stuffy feeling, an air of anticipation.

Adults are there, but they are only shadowy figures in unaccustomed clothing. They are talking to her, but she doesn't hear them. She walks through the adjoining room, through a kind of bridal arch of doorways. It seems to go on forever, like a tunnel. At the end is the lighted window facing out on the street, with its lace curtains. Beneath the window is the coffin. It is open. And in front of the coffin is a little stool.

She knows that the stool is for the grown-ups. She sees her father kneeling in his black suit on it, facing into the coffin. He turns and she sees the tears running down his cheeks—the first and only time. He cries out in Italian, and some other shadows come and rush him off.

She walks calmly to the stool and, instead of kneeling, she stands up on it to see what is inside.

It is her mother. She is lying so peaceful, so quiet. Her face, although waxy and strange, still bears a tinge of youth. And, strangest of all, she has on her wedding gown.

Christine feels nothing, nothing at all, neither sadness nor pain. Just curiosity: why is she wearing her wedding gown, which hung in the closet of her mother's bedroom for so long? She is going to God, they told her. Is she marrying God?

Why did she die? The grown-ups whisper. She had seen her mother in the old Samaritan Hospital, when she had pleaded with her father to help her jump out the window. The pain, she had said. The pain. The last time she had seen her mother she had been trying to put on lipstick. Her hand shook and the lipstick went on crooked. She looked like a clown, Christine thought, and she laughed and even her mother laughed, although Chris could tell she wasn't really happy.

"It's gone to her liver," the relatives whispered. "It's gone

to the bones. Into the brain. It's all over," they said, "all over."
    She died in the house.
    Her father grabs her from behind and lifts her off the stool by her elbows. Christine struggles. She wants to see her mother in her dress one more time.
    "That's it," says her father, gruffly. "Time to go to church. Can't keep God waiting."
    And around her all the old aunts, the old relatives, smelling of powder, are whispering.

Strong checked the mimeo sheet on the wall. He was scrubbing with Wolf, a third-year resident.
    "Where the hell is Wolf?" he yelled, in the kind of bravado style affected in operating rooms.
    "Where did that cucumber go?" the head nurse, Anne-Marie, echoed angrily. Anne-Marie looked really menacing that morning, her mousy hair caught up in a tight bun, her eyes swimming behind their thick bottom-of-the-bottle lenses.
    Wolf waved a hand from across the corridor.
    "Hi, Wolf, how are you?" Strong said. Wolf was a third-year resident, but he was older than most. He had had to repeat medical school in the United States when the authorities refused to accept his East European degree. He was also a know-it-all.
    A medical student was standing in on the operation. She was sweet looking—at least she was from the bridge of her nose up to her hairline. The rest of her was obscured by her surgical mask. She had soft brown eyes and long, long eyelashes. She stood by the side of the table, where Christine was now stretched out, an orange tube in her mouth. The student's hands were pursed together in what might have been an unconscious attitude of prayer. Strong wondered momentarily if she was going to pass out on him during the operation. That had happened to him once.
    "What medical school are you from?" Strong asked.
    "I go to school in the Caribbean," said the student.
    "Where'd you do your undergraduate work?"
    "At Barnard."
    Strong shook his head angrily. "It's disgusting that they force American kids from good schools to go down there and pay a fortune instead of making places for them here."

"The conditions aren't too good," said the student. "Constant blackouts and so forth. It's very primitive."

"Well, I'll try to teach you a few things while you're up here."

Suddenly Anne-Marie, the head nurse, piped up. "I want everybody to stop talking in here or we'll be here all day. It takes too long to get anything done."

She was rude and out of line, and Strong could have easily put her in his place. Talking in the operating room was useful and important: it kept things moving smoothly. Coordinating a dozen people to do *anything* was difficult under the best of circumstances. Coordinating an operation, where a life could hang in the balance, required a great deal of tact as well as discipline.

Strong could have taken this remark up with the head of surgery or with the director of nursing, but he chose to ignore it. Everyone had the right to a bad day now and then. And surgeons depended on the scrub nurses to have things ready for them when they operate, to make the operation run without hitches.

Most laypeople had the idea that surgeons were gods or tyrants in the operating room. That was good for TV, but in reality it was a bit more complicated, as every resident soon learned. There was politics in the operating room as everywhere else.

The room was quiet now except for the "ping ping ping" of the physio-control machine, punctuated by an occasional bullfrog noise. The anesthesiologist had left the mechanism in the hands of his resident, who sat attentively, squeezing the black bag. Christine was carefully disrobed, and then Strong ordered the placement of sheets.

"Can I have some more sheets?" he yelled.

No one answered. Anne-Marie was not to be seen—she was in the adjoining room watching the autoclave, a kind of pressure cooker for instruments.

"Hello. This is earth calling—God knows where."

Still no response.

"And this is the person complaining that I go too slow," he said to the medical student. " 'I talk—we're slow.' That's projection, basic psychiatry."

The head nurse finally emerged with some blue sheets,

which were now draped to cover Christine's whole body. Even her face was shielded from the operation by a sheet positioned about six inches above her nose. They had taped her eyelids shut.

Only her breasts were exposed, glistening red-orange from the disinfectant in the intense sunlight of the surgical lamp. The resident, Wolf, wiped them dry and now they were ready, just the two mammary glands left exposed in a sea of bright blue.

Strong and the resident conferred on the tumors.

According to Strong, there were three tumors: two in the left breast and one in the right. The resident, on the other hand, claimed there were two in each breast. There was nothing Strong dreaded more than missing a tumor that needed excision, but, on the other hand, he hated the idea of unnecessary surgery.

"This one and this one makes two," Strong said, feeling the left breast. "Then this one here," he said, touching the chest wall of the right breast, "makes three."

The resident still dickered. "What about this?"

"That's a lipoma," said Strong, feeling it. "It's soft. We're not going to make an incision for that."

Strong nodded to the resident to begin. Although many patients are chagrined to learn that their operations might have been performed by a resident instead of the surgeon whom they are paying, this was often inevitable. Surgeons must have assistants during the operation—to hold the retractors, to tie off bleeders, and to be generally a second pair of hands. In addition, if there are to be more surgeons, then obviously they must get their hands-on experience somewhere. Abuse creeps in when an occasional "ghost" surgeon simply leaves the surgery to his resident and goes off to have a cup of coffee or perform another operation. Strong, on the other hand, did everything but physically guide the hand of the assistant.

"No, no, no," he yelled, as Wolf began his incision. "How are you doing that? Transverse! Make a straight line right across."

The resident drew the scalpel across the flesh as indicated. Dark red blood welled up from the wound.

"Retraction," Strong said. He turned and took the gloved hand of the young medical student, who was looking a bit queasy.

"What's your name?" he asked her.
"Katherine."
"Katherine, here, hold this," he said, handing her a kind of fork, the other end of which was in the woman's breast. She held it gingerly. Wolf made as if to cut. "Stop," said Strong. "You have to be able to show me breast tissue that is tumor. You don't just remove fat. That makes a much larger hole than necessary. *This* is the tumor right here." With his own retractor he pointed to a piece of tissue, subtly different from the surrounding area.

"Try not to cut before I clamp," he added, "or else we'll be looking for bleeders all the live-long day."

"Go ahead," he said. The resident's problem was that he wasn't cutting in the demarcated area along a transverse plane, but digging into the tissue. This would sever new veins and arteries that hadn't been tied off yet or sealed by the electric Bovie knife.

"Right across the top. If you cut that way, it's going to bleed down there and then I have *tsurris*. You understand *tsurris*? Aggravation."

There were eight instruments in the tiny wound now—clamps, knives, retractors. Katherine, the medical student, suddenly had a weird image of the patient as a bull in a bullring and the surgical instruments, which dangled from her, as banderillas. She quickly chased the image from her mind.

They had removed the first tumor now.

"It's all out," he said, with satisfaction. "Let's 'buzz' this."

The resident applied the Bovie knife, which cauterized the bleeding arteries. The green electrosurgical unit made a racket.

Strong stuck his finger in the wound. "Excellent. This is very good. We've got nothing left in there."

He glanced briefly at the monitor as the patient missed a heartbeat. Then it steadied itself:

>mean arterial pressure .109
>heart rate BPM 090
>systolic pressure 109
>diastolic pressure 053

He glanced at the anesthesiology resident, who didn't look up. Everything was okay.

The wound was still oozing blood. Wolf seemed hell-bent

on sewing it up. "It's very embarrassing after surgery to have a blood clot under there," he said. "Give me some more juice on the coag, please."

The resident proceeded to sew up the wound with black thread. The cut was too small to require staples.

Strong turned to the medical student.

"So what tumors of the breast do you take out?" he asked.

"All suspicious lesions that do not disappear upon aspiration."

"Good," said Strong. "Can't we just use a mammogram?"

"No, it only tells you where it is," she said, although it came out more as a question than an answer.

"If we feel the tumor do we still do a mammogram?"

"Yes."

"Why?"

"Because there may be others we don't feel."

"Good girl," he said, "Sorry, that is correct. I didn't mean to be sexist. More co-ag," he yelled suddenly.

"Doctor," said the head nurse. "Do you want this specimen sent down?"

"Frozen," said Strong, indicating a frozen section. "But wait till we have all the specimens."

They were starting in on the second tumor, also in the left breast.

"Damn it to hell," said the resident. He had lost control of the knife momentarily.

"Why don't you take a fifteen blade?" said Strong. "It makes it easier to control your incision."

This was particularly humiliating to Wolf, who felt and acted like the big kid unfairly put back in kindergarten.

"Find that tumor," said Strong. "That's the name of the game."

Wolf couldn't. He kept trying to cut normal tissue.

"Raise the table a little bit," said Strong. Since he was taller than his resident that had a subtle meaning to all: the doctor was taking charge. And since Strong would have to rate Wolf, and all the residents on his team, at the end of the month, it was a bad omen for the young expert.

"This is it, I got it," Strong said, after a moment. He used his scalpel to make a sharp incision at the base of the waxy yellow tumor. "Very good. That takes care of number two." He dropped it into the stainless-steel tray.

"What about micro-calcification?" he asked Katherine. This was a particularly elusive form of growth that could not be felt under normal circumstances.

"They show up on mammograms as little white dots," said Katherine.

"What is the incidence of cancer in micro-calcification?" he asked, enjoying the chance to teach. He had taught for years at Brooklyn-Cumberland Medical Center, an affiliate of Downstate Medical School, and missed it now that he had gone into private practice.

The student hesitated. "I don't know," she said, worried.

"It's high. About twenty-five to thirty percent. And remember: even two or three calcification dots on a mammogram can indicate cancer."

Strong proceeded to run Katherine through the latest techniques in diagnosis such as diaphinography, or transillumination of the breast with a special lamp. All the while he kept his eyes on the resident's suturing. He wasn't entirely pleased: there was a little tear in one corner of the incision. Sloppiness. "Careful what you do," he said. "Take special care with that corner."

"The breast isn't so important," said the anesthesiologist's resident.

"To me it is!" Strong said, in an unusual display of anger.

"Are you the husband?" asked the resident slyly.

"It matters to me," said Strong, "and I want this to look good." He knew that his word-of-mouth reputation among women rested in good measure on the smallness and neatness of his cuts. Many times the biopsy scars were almost invisible one year later.

"The husband doesn't even care. He doesn't look at that," said the resident, implying that a husband only cares about one thing.

"This husband does," said Strong. "He told me specifically he wanted her breasts to look good."

"He probably cares more about the breasts than about the tumor. What would he do if it turned out to be cancer? He should be so lucky to get away with a few little scars."

They had sewn up the two incisions on the left breast and were getting ready to do the right breast.

"Here, let me do this one," said Strong. "I haven't done any surgery for three days and my fingers are falling off." Lately, it seemed all the basic cutting had been performed by his resident staff.

As he cut, daubed, and cauterized, he actually started humming gently. The portrait of a man happy with his work.

He had removed the tumor deftly and assigned it to the little steel tray in about half the time it would have taken the resident. The cut was small and neat, the bleeding totally under control from the start.

It was a knobby little thing, about a centimeter in diameter.

Nobody gave it much of a glance. "Adenoma," said the resident, and Strong nodded: a very unremarkable-looking benign growth. Standing back, he allowed the resident to sew up the final incision.

Strong walked off, washed his hands, removed his surgical cap and hat. He chatted with another of his residents, who wrote the name of a special patient he was supposed to visit in pen right on his green hospital pants. Strong ambled through the corridor and got himself a glass of milk from the refrigerator in the anesthesiologists' lounge.

He had a ton of phone calls to make but first he would visit Christine, who would be stirring back to life about now. But he decided to call pathology first, just in case.

He got the pathologist on the phone. "This is Dr. Strong. I'm calling about those three specimens I just sent." A pause. "Wait a second." His eyelashes batting. "Are you talking about —I gave you a right breast. Specimen Number Three was *what*? What kind of . . . *What* is it?"

He stood there for a moment, in the corner of the recovery room, his lips puffed out slightly, his fingers to his forehead as if in pain.

"Holy shit," he said, finally, quietly. "Left breast is benign. You're sure about that. The third one is *not* an adenoma. Where are you now?" he asked. He could see that Christine was stirring already. "I'm coming down to you."

The pathology department was on the second floor. He smelled the formaldehyde as soon as he got off the elevator. To the uninitiated, it was more than a bit bizarre. Grisly specimens of human organs lay in bottles, a bit helter-skelter on the shelves. Textbooks, well-thumbed, lay open on the bench, stained by chemicals. Autopsies were taking place in the room next door. Reports. Case records. Plastic trays filled with plastic cups with obscene human fragments in them. Yet the pathologists seemed unaffected by all this gore.

At the center of this scene sat a large man and his microscope. He was a regular bear of a man, about as charming looking as a Russian general. But he was a fine pathologist who rarely made mistakes.

"This is a mucin-producing tumor, Strong," he said bluntly.

"Cancer? This is not benign? Are you sure?"

"Mucinous carcinoma."

"This is a thirty-five-year-old woman," Strong said, his face reflecting his shock.

"You've had younger ones," the pathologist reminded him.

"I know, but this looked and felt just like an adenoma. This is very rare. But the prognosis on these mucin-producers is good, isn't it?"

"Well, I wouldn't say 'good.' Let's just say it's *less bad.* But it's definitely cancer."

Suddenly Strong was seized with fear: What if they were wrong? It just didn't seem possible. Maybe there had been a slipup—it happened, even in the best of hospitals—and somebody else's tumor got mixed up with Christine's.

"Let me see it," he said suddenly.

The pathologist didn't object but fished around and came up with a plastic cup, similar to the kind pills are packed in at the pharmacy.

One glance and Strong said, "That is it." It was the same one that Strong had taken out of her fifteen minutes before. Unbelievable.

"They're peculiar. The cells are surrounded with a mucous-like substance. It's unusual, Strong. I've seen one or two of these in collection. But we haven't had a live one since I don't know how long."

"I can't believe this," Strong said, holding his head.

"Believe it," the pathologist said, twisting his bullish neck to cradle the phone.

"How am I going to tell her?" he asked.

The pathologist was speaking into the mouthpiece, onto another case already. He didn't go in for formalities such as hello and good-bye.

"How the hell do you tell a woman something like this?" Strong repeated, to no one in particular.

Chris lay on the bed in the recovery room. The world was white. She was dreaming, a flow of light waving past her face like silk banners. Banners floating on the wind. As she floated upward they came into focus and she realized what they were: the multicolored jerseys of the runners in the marathon. Soon the world was all primary colors, of a brilliance and purity she had not seen since she was a little girl. Lollipop colors, the colors of the little alphabet blocks her grandmother had given her.

Then she was awake. The world was white again. Women in white shuffled past her. One came over, peered into her face, and disappeared. She struggled to get free, but couldn't. She tried to cry out, but nothing emerged. She lay like that for a long time, until she no longer felt like struggling.

A hospital. She was in a hospital.

There was a sign. She struggled to read it, but it oozed away from her each time she got close. A picture of a little boy, a cute little black child. Letter by letter she pieced it together, although it seemed to take an eternity.

> *I know I'm*
> *somebody*
> *'cause God don't*
> *make no junk!!*

What did it mean? She faded out again. When she awoke again there was a man standing by her bedside and she knew who he was.

"Christine," said Dr. Strong.

"What happened?" she asked.

"Christine," he said. "I'm sorry. But it didn't turn out like we hoped. Two of the tumors were benign, but the one in the right breast was cancer." She moaned.

"I hate to have to tell you this, dear, but I think you have to know the truth."

"Don't tell me that," she cried, her eyes widening with fear. She didn't cry, but she whimpered, as if in extreme physical pain. "Don't tell me that."

"I'm sorry. I have to." He paused, looking away. "It was an unusual type of tumor. I'll explain it all to you later. I didn't want to leave you here in suspense, Chris, without knowing."

She licked her lips nervously. They felt like parchment.

"Unusual in what way?" she asked, trying to be interested, dispassionate, detached.

"I'll explain it to you. It's—"

"What did you do?" she interrupted. She was seized with a sudden panic. She thought, Oh, my God! They've removed my breasts!

"I removed the tumor, that's all. It was about one centimeter in size." He held up his thumb and forefinger to indicate that small growth.

She started sobbing now. At least she had her breast. Without realizing it, she reached out and placed her hand on top of his on the sidebars of her bed, groaning as if her guts were wrenching inside her.

There was silence. A nurse looked on with pity from where she was making up another bed.

"But I feel good," Chris whispered.

"I know you feel good," said Strong. He couldn't believe it. The fact that she was a runner, a serious type who did five to ten miles a day, deeply impressed him. He tried to do his two miles every morning along the F.D.R. Drive, but not always with the greatest success.

"How can this be?"

"It was a very small, localized thing. It looked just like a benign gland, a fibroadenoma. It was the one on the right side, the one you discovered first."

Suddenly she started shaking, nothing violent, but involuntary and alarming all the same. She thought of John and what his reaction might be.

"You didn't remove anything else?"

"I only have permission to do a biopsy," he said, and he sounded like a man who took such agreements very seriously indeed. "We'll have to talk. It will take about an hour. I'll sit down with you and your husband and we'll discuss the alternatives." Pause. Now comes the hard part. "You're going to need more treatment to the right breast."

She seemed puzzled. More treatment? What did that mean? It could mean anything. But at least she would have time to think.

"I will present you and your husband with a very good plan," he said.

Basically, if only that one breast were involved, and if none of the lymph nodes was positive, Christine would have a choice: she could go for the modified radical, or she could have quadrant resection with radiation of the breast. In either case she could be reconstructed after six months, since chemotherapy probably would not be required. Part of it would depend on what she found out about her mother's death. If her mother had died of breast cancer then she would have a greater chance herself of a recurrence. In that case she might opt for a modified radical. He would explain all this to them when they came in to see him.

"I feel trapped," she said suddenly, gasping loudly.

"What do you mean?" he asked.

"I can't get up," she said.

"You're not supposed to run a marathon."

It was strange, Strong thought: she had articulated the very word that was going through his own mind—they were all trapped by a murdering disease that so monstrously cut down young and "healthy" women like this in their prime. He was fighting an enemy in the dark, his tiny scalpel against the scythe.

"Do you think you got it all?" The classic question. But instead of the storybook answer, Strong had to tell her: "The entire tumor was removed, but I don't know if that tumor has spread or metastasized to other parts of your body." With her bias against further therapy, he just couldn't allow her the luxury of false optimism.

"I don't want to be melodramatic," she said, "but I don't want to die of cancer."

He wanted to say something—that it would be all right, that he would take care of everything. It was so tempting to give out with the bullshit right now, so easy for himself and for the patient. Instead, he simply squeezed her hand, looked into her eyes for a moment, in order to share her fear and pain, and then walked like a burdened man to the bank of elevators.

As Strong left the recovery room after seeing Christine Mackin, the nurse at the desk came running after him. She caught him in the hall. "Call the pathologist," she said.

Strong went down to the physicians' lounge to call the pathologist. If he tells me now he's made a mistake, I'll kill him, he thought. I'll positively kill him.

The pathologist had more bad news. "Don't tell me," Strong said, literally pulling on his gray hair. "Don't tell me this. There's atypical cells in the left breast. Right, right, right. Paraffin section Wednesday. May be bilateral cancer. Damn!" He hung up. They would have to wait for the definitive pathological tests. But if the pathologist thought he saw atypical cells upon frozen-section examination, he would probably find them on paraffin as well. This changed the whole picture. He remembered a phrase from the textbook about these mucin-producing tumors. Bilateral cancer in both breasts or spread to other areas "materially darken the prognosis."

Damn, damn, damn.

"What's-a-matter, Strong?"

It was Greenfeld,* a urologist.

"How's the urine business, Greenfeld?" Strong asked. His face, voice, and whole manner showed his distress, however.

"Lose one?" asked Greenfeld.

"Can you imagine?" said Strong. "Thirty-five years old. Breast cancer. It looked like a typical adenoma. Felt like a typical adenoma."

"But it warn't no typical adenoma, eh?"

"Mucinous carcinoma." He paused. He didn't really want to confide in this relative stranger. And yet he felt the pressing need to reach out to someone, to talk it out.

"Sometimes I wonder what the hell I'm doing," said Strong. "I mean, it gets worse and worse. I had a young girl in here a couple of months ago with breast cancer."

"Well, take it easy," said Greenfeld, obviously uncomfort-

*Name changed.

able with the drift of the conversation. He ambled out, a stack of records almost a foot thick under his arm.

Strong pulled one of the phones over to his chair and dialed. It was Christine's home number. He had looked for her husband in the waiting room and had him paged, but he was nowhere to be found. Maybe he just doesn't want to know, thought Strong. That sometimes happened. Husbands and lovers and even parents copped out at the last minute. Well, if that's the case, the hell with him, he thought angrily. He's going to know, he's got to share in this. The phone rang and rang. The husband meanwhile was wandering around the hospital looking for Dr. Strong, and didn't hear the page. He was equally angry at the doctor.

Suddenly the lounge felt very oppressive. It was simply business as usual for the rest of the world. The comfortable armchairs, the old pictures of long-gone house staffs, the carefree conversations of the other doctors. It was hard for Strong to understand how this young woman could have cancer and yet nothing changed. The world, as they said, did not come to an end.

"There are three big shots in thoracic surgery. . . ."

". . . convention in Hawaii next year. A meeting is good for you to know what's going on. . . ."

"I've been to Hawaii already."

"Dr. Strong, nine-four-three-six. Dr. Strong, nine-four-three-six." The page operator interrupted his reverie. He called his service. One of his patients in Manhattan had started hemorrhaging and was being admitted to the emergency room. Strong grabbed his jacket and ran to the exit. He could be at Beth Israel in half an hour, God and traffic willing.

There was something she had to know.

All her life she had heard these whispered rumors, but Christine had never really found out exactly what had happened to her mother. Now she had a medical reason to do so—Dr. Strong needed to know. She remembered her mother in the hospital—Samaritan—on President Street between Fifth and Sixth Avenues. Christine thought perhaps she could get some medical information from the hospital her mother had been in, some facts that could illuminate that period of her life and explain her current problems. But, to her amazement and dismay, the hospital was gone: the building had been converted to a co-op. She wondered briefly from which window her mother had asked her father to help her jump during the last agonizing moments of her life. Probably that one with the ferns and Gro-Lite in the window, she thought ironically. Life goes on, and eventually all traces of mother, father, children disappear. She hurried away, back to her brownstone, to John and to Melanie.

And so there was nothing to do but go visit her father. He was living in a house on the fringe of the Carroll Gardens neighborhood in which she had grown up. He worked part-time in a local shoe repair shop, and had retired early on Social Security. His heart wasn't good.

"Ah, so you've come back," said her father when he saw her.

"Hi, Dad," she said, kissing him on the cheek. "Where's Jeannie? Did I miss her?" Jeannie was her father's current wife. Chris felt a deep resentment toward her, but all the same tried to be civil.

"Bingo," said her father. "Everything okay with you?"

Her natural impulse to that question was to say "sure," and it took a deliberate effort to say, "No, Pop. It's not okay. I have to go in for an operation next week." Her voice quivered as she said it. How she hated that quiver!

"Operation, huh? You look okay."

"They say I've got a tumor, Dad. In my breast."

"Gee, that's too bad. Really." He didn't seem awfully upset, though. "You know, it sounds crazy, but I won't even be around next week. I'm going home—to Italy, I mean—just next week. I think I told you. It's been planned for a long time. I'd lose the money if I canceled now. . . ."

"Sure, I understand. But actually, I didn't come for sympathy. I'm trying to find out some details of our family's history. In particular, I'd like to know about Momma. What was wrong with her? What she died of."

"Yeah, well, in those days you didn't talk about things like that. You kept it to yourself. But she had it, too. Cancer. Breast cancer. I guess this kind of thing sort of runs in families."

It wasn't a complete surprise to Christine, of course, but still, hearing it outright like this gave her chills.

Her father went on: "It's in the family, all right. Both her sisters—you remember Carmelina and that other one—they both had it."

"And what about Grandma?"

"Come to think of it, she had it too. Gee, I'm really sorry about this. But it's in the blood and so there's nothing that can be done about it. It's just, well, fate."

The news was bad, worse that she had expected. She wanted to get home, cuddle up with John, and hear his consoling words. She wanted to call Strong and have him tell her, "Well, it really doesn't matter that much. With modern medical techniques we can defy fate. There's no such thing as fate. There's only our knowledge or ignorance of the disease."

She had a sudden feeling of suffocation here, followed by a surge of anger toward her father. He was never there for her when she needed him. This trip to Italy had sure come at a convenient time. She grabbed her bag and stood up to go.

"Well, I'm sorry for you," said her father. "Sorry I can't be there. But I'll be back in three weeks and I tell you what. I'll bring you back something. A present, something really swell from Italy."

"Yeah, that's great," said Christine, and she fled into the cold night air of the Brooklyn winter.

Christine's impending operation and the need to make a decision about the course of treatment had thrown the whole house into confusion. She pondered the alternatives. On the one hand, there had been some good news. The cells in her other breast were not "atypical" upon paraffin section—the pathologist's first impression, upon frozen section, had been pessimistic. This meant that a quadrant resection was a real possibility. And the advantages of the more sparing procedure were obvious: three-quarters of the breast would remain, and the rest could be reconstructed in six months.

On the other hand, the fact that her mother and so many other relatives had died of breast cancer worried her. Breast cancer, Strong had explained, was multifocal in origin. There was always a chance of it returning to the affected breast despite the radiation that would be directed to that portion of the body following a quadrant resection.

She was nervous and on edge, and it was affecting her carefully nurtured relationship with her eleven-year-old daughter, Melanie. This crisis coincided with that peculiar pre-adolescent age in which kids can be brutally outspoken toward their parents.

She and John tried not to talk about what was going to happen in front of her, but Melanie was smart and overheard their conversations.

The weekend before Christine was due to enter the hospital for the operation she was in the bathroom, drying off after a shower. Melanie, as was her wont, burst into the bathroom looking for her brush, and before she knew it was directly in front of her mother's breasts. The biopsy scar was uncovered and although it was minor—especially compared to what was about to come—it was a terrible harbinger.

Melanie screamed, "Ooooh! Ooooh!" like she had just seen something filthy and disgusting. And this was for just the biopsy scar, a small red line or two. Imagine what her reaction would be to the mastectomy, even the quadrantectomy!

That Monday Chris took her to school. Melanie was walking with her friend Claudia; the two of them looked cute with their matching oversized Danish bookbags. Claudia was her best friend, and she had told her about her mother's operation. "I need somebody to talk to," she had said, with that almost unnatural maturity of the eleven-year-old. "I need to let them know that I'm scared and that I feel hurt."

Chris let her, although she didn't relish the thought of the word getting out to all the parents. That was an emotional thing —trying to hide the obvious. But sooner or later it would get out.

"I think you're a bad mother," Melanie had said suddenly, as they turned onto her school block.

"Don't say that," Chris said, cringing. "Anything you want to know, you can always come to Daddy and me. Ask us anything, anything."

"I'm mad at you."

"Why? What did I do?"

"Why didn't you take good care of yourself? You should have gone to doctors. You didn't take care of yourself."

She ran ahead and Claudia followed.

Chris tried to object: she had gone to the doctor as soon as she found it. But in a deeper sense—and this is what hurt so bad—she wondered if Melanie hadn't hit on the truth. For she had never deliberately examined herself. As stupid as it now seemed, she always relied on John to examine her breasts for her—during sex play, "wrestling," as she called it. Now that seemed so ridiculous: it wasn't good sex for a man to be doing a breast examination while he was feeling you up! Nor was it good medicine, for such an exam was sloppy and hasty at best.

But what had happened to her mother had scared her. She didn't intend to be another victim if she could help it. And here she was, despite her ostrich attitude, in the same position as her mother. Hopefully, with better treatment today, she might survive a lot longer than her mother had.

Melanie had disappeared, and Chris became panicky for a moment. Then she emerged from the old-fashioned candy store next door to the school. She had a Baby Ruth and a frozen Mars bar sticking out of her sack.

"Come here, young lady," said Chris, trying to assert her authority. "You know you're not allowed to eat candy in school and especially in the morning."

"This is for after lunch," Melanie said, enunciating each and every syllable icily.

Chris put her hand on her daughter's shoulder. "Honey, you know I feel sorry about this."

Her daughter looked at her directly. Tears were welling up quickly in Melanie's eyes. "If you're not going to live, then I don't want to live," she said, quavering.

Her friend Claudia's eyes also began to water over.

Chris was speechless. Melanie broke away and ran toward the school. Chris let her go—she needed to go to school. At least there she could take her mind off her problem. But deep inside she wanted to run after her, to stop her, hug her, make it right. If only there was some way to make this disaster right.

Mildred

It had been a wonderful afternoon. Carol Rosenbloom's Head Start group had behaved themselves beautifully. There were twelve and by law there had to be six adults with them. At the last minute, she had been able to convince only four parents to accompany the trip. That had left one opening. She had called her mother, Mildred, who gladly accepted the assignment to be a mother for the afternoon to two pre-schoolers.

They had seen the Hall of Minerals, and the kids had run eagerly from one brightly lit display to another. They had admired the mastedons and the dinosaurs, of course, and finished it off with tolerable hot dogs and mushy sauerkraut in the cafeteria. Then when the first child threw the first serious temper tantrum, they knew it was time to go home. Back to Brooklyn, back to Canarsie.

As they were emerging from the museum, on the sidewalk within the shadow of Teddy Roosevelt, Mildred Rosenbloom slipped on an unseen patch of ice and went down.

"Ma, are you all right?" Carol screamed.

When she was able to talk—which itself took a minute or two—she said, "I'm all right. Boy, I really hurt my knee, though." She felt the knee this way and that. It didn't feel broken.

"Are you sure?" Carol was almost in a panic.

"I'm sure," said Mildred, wincing in pain. "If there was anything broken I'm sure I'd know from it." She leaned against the heavy iron fence. "That doesn't mean it doesn't hurt, though," she added. Carol picked up her umbrella. It was a big cotton-and-wood thing, a present brought back from Europe by a neighbor.

"Thank you, dear," she said. "And this damn umbrella gave me a good *zetz* in the boobie," she added, looking at it angrily.

"Thank God you're all right," said Carol. The children, who had been standing around looking precociously concerned, now started to break away and get back into their games.

"Watch the kids, Carol. Your mother can take care of herself. She's a tough old bird."

Carol leaned over and kissed her mother. Despite the fact that she was now married herself and lived miles away, the two of them were still extraordinarily close. In some ways, the relationship was the most important one Carol had. People sometimes made fun of her for this—called Mildred a "Jewish mother" and all that. But for her, the love of her mother was something warm, generous, and wonderful in an otherwise selfish world.

It was a few months later, in the spring, that Mildred first noticed it. She had been bathing, getting herself ready for Phil. They had always enjoyed each other, but to their wonder and amazement, love had only gotten *better* for them with age. They had had kids early in life. It was when their children had grown up and gone out on their own, and they had finally discovered the meaning of the word "privacy," that their lovemaking had matured and blossomed. It was funny—not at all the way things were "supposed to be" when she was growing up. As a child she had thought of sex as something very romantic. So romantic, in fact, that she thought only very beautiful people could engage in it. Her ignorance at marriage was abysmal. When she had children, therefore, she had tried to explain the facts of life to them in a sober, scientific way, the way mothers of the Dr. Spock era used to do. Her son Steven had startled her when he said, "Then you and Daddy have had sex *twice*, right, Mommy?" She had obviously forgotten to tell the kids one important fact about lovemaking—the pleasure. And, in a way, it was only now, in their mature years, that she and Phil had discovered it fully for themselves.

She was reaching for the talcum powder on the top shelf of the bathroom when she saw it. It was in the same place where the umbrella had struck her outside the museum. It had left a black and blue mark then, but that had gone away. Now there was something else there. It was poking up from the surface of the upper breast as she stretched her arm. She gingerly put her hand to it: it was hot and hard.

She felt it carefully and caught a glimpse of her frightened face in the mirror. She turned away.

Mildred knew what she should do: enough of her friends in Canarsie had been through this that she was no stranger to breast problems. She should get herself to a doctor, tell Phil, tell the children. Have it taken care of, before it took care of her. But, as she stood with her hand on the doorknob, she knew she couldn't follow her own good advice.

Problems . . . her daughter's job difficulties, her son's impending divorce, her son-in-law's unemployment. How could she put them all through *this* now? Why did it have to happen to me, when everyone is depending on me to be the strong one? No, cancer or no cancer, she thought, it would have to wait. For the others' sake. And what about the trip to Israel that she and Phil had been planning for twenty years? Now that they were semi-retired, they had a chance to go and the money to enjoy themselves. Instead they should spend the money on hospitals and doctors? It seemed impossible, ridiculous. She would just wait, and hope that things would improve. Sometimes these things just went away.

That evening in bed, Phil was his usual enthusiastic self. She pushed him away when he wanted to touch her there.

"What's wrong?" he asked, his intuition fine-tuned to her moods and needs.

"Oh, it's nothing," she lied. "It's just . . . that I'm still sore there from the black and blue mark, the fall outside the museum."

"That was a while ago," he said. "Maybe you should have it looked at." But they went on to other things, and that was the last he mentioned it. Perhaps he would never notice.

Christine

At night Christine and her husband lay in the dark in their bedroom. They lay for a long time without speaking while he held her hand.

"What should I do?" she asked finally. "Strong wants a decision by tomorrow. I can't put it off any longer."

"You once said you would never have a mastectomy," he reminded her.

"That was for you," she said.

"For me?"

"I didn't want you to have to live with . . . an incomplete woman."

He laughed, more out of surprise than any feeling of amusement. "That's what you think of me? That I care about things like that? It's *you* I'm after, not your breast. I love *you*, don't you understand? Any decision you make has got to be based on what's safest. I don't care about the cosmetic part. Besides, didn't Strong say they could probably reconstruct?"

"Yes," she answered, almost in a whisper. "I could still have the quadrantectomy," she said. "They would just take out the tumor and some surrounding tissue. But it would leave me almost intact."

"I don't know," John said slowly. "It's kind of new, isn't it?"

"A lot of people are having it done. One of the other patients showed me an article in a magazine."

"I'm sure they're right," said John. "But what concerns me is your safety. If you'll be as comfortable with that quadrantectomy as with the bigger operation, if you feel it's just as safe, then I guess you should do it. But if you're always going to harbor doubts and fears, then it might be worth the sacrifice of the breast." He paused. What he didn't want to do was make up her mind for her. This was *her* decision. He knew eventually she would come up with the answer that was best for her. "Whatever you do," he said finally, "is okay with me. Just so long as you get well." Christine raised his hand to her face and held it there until they both fell asleep.

In the end, Christine opted for the modified radical. The idea of living constantly with the fear of cancer returning to the affected breast was just too much for her. Also, deep down she was a very conservative person, and although the lumpectomies and quadrantectomies were more and more common, to her they were still very new and therefore suspect.

Strong explained to her that they would have to watch her very carefully after the operation, with frequent and close examinations. Cancer often appeared in the opposite breast, especially in a woman like Christine who had already had benign tumors there.

She had spent eight days in the hospital, and it seemed an even longer period. Walking among people had already become unfamiliar, and the street seemed incredibly bright, noisy, and gritty. It was equally strange to be back in the house on Montgomery Street. Everything was solid, the same, yet it all had an unreal quality to it.

"What a mess," she said, looking over the first floor of the brownstone. "I'd better get to work." The Mackins had bought this brownstone the year before and were renovating it slowly. John had tried to explain to her the resulting tax benefits, but she never could understand him. All she knew was that there was a perpetual commotion. In addition, John was no housekeeper. The kitchen was piled high with TV-dinner debris.

"I've got to get in there," she said with determination.

"Let it lie," he said, pressing her hand. "You're incredible.

If you were on your way to a concentration camp I really believe you'd make 'em wait so you could tidy up the house first." She laughed. "You keep the chemical companies of America in business, singlehandedly. Take it easy. Right now there's more important business, anyway."

He went off into the kitchen, and Christine started to unpack. How wonderful it felt to be home again. Melanie would be home, too, in a few hours, and then they would all be together again. A family, a real family. She couldn't believe it.

"What's this?" she asked, as he emerged through the louvered doors.

"Tom Vargas sent it over," he said, holding up a bottle of champagne. Tom was a neighbor in whom John had confided about their problems. It was the Spanish type—economical but expensive tasting. "He sends you his love. So, shall we?" Without waiting for a reply, John worked the cork up with his two thumbs, and it popped loudly—such a happy, domestic, nonmedical sound. He had brought out two of their crystal glasses and poured her a smoking glassful.

"To you, my darling," he said.

"To you, you sentimental slob," she said, clinking glasses. It was delicious.

John came over and put his arms around her.

"Well, I'm going to get unpacked, and then I'm going to try and take a bath. You know, that's one of the worst things about the hos—"

"I sort of had different plans," he said in a low voice.

She couldn't quite believe her ears. "What? What do you mean?"

"I had different plans for this afternoon," he said, smiling and running his hands over her shoulders.

She pulled back. "God, you've got to be kidding, John. You mean *now*?" She gasped, out of breath. "I don't know. I've got so much to deal with. Too much. I mean . . . I feel so ugly."

"You're not ugly," he whispered, running his hand down her arm.

"And I'm so . . . I don't know. It's all so strange. I just got out of the hospital! I mean, I want to keep you happy, but . . ."

John sat down on the couch. "That's okay," he said, trying to sound understanding.

"Are you sure?" she asked. She felt terrible. It was all so sudden and surprising, though. She had pictured in her mind a long period of adjustment, a kind of halting approach toward each other, with some possibly terrible consequences along the way. And now, they weren't in the house five minutes, and he wanted to make love to her!

"I don't feel right, John. I mean, my hair's greasy, I've got one tit. . . ."

He laughed uproariously. "And what the hell difference does *that* make? I love you."

She looked at him for a long moment. She wanted him, too, she realized, but it was her mental attitude that was keeping her back. Then, suddenly, something inside melted. "Oh, what the hell!" she said almost lightheartedly.

John laughed happily. Holding the champagne in one hand, he led her up the steep stairs with the other. She could tell from his determined manner that the horny so-and-so had been planning this all week long.

"Are you sure . . . you want to do this?" she asked as they reached the bedroom. She didn't know exactly what to do. Normally she would have quickly thrown her clothes over the chair, because making love to John was her greatest pleasure in life. But now she felt a peculiar strangeness with her own husband. They both knew what the problem was, of course.

"Sure, I'm sure. Why should there be any difference? There *isn't* any difference. I've been waiting for you for such a long, long time." It had only been eight days, but it did feel like a long time indeed. She unbuttoned her blouse hesitantly and turned her back to him as she took it off.

"Do you want to show me?" he asked.

She had lain awake in the hospital bed thinking, wondering about this very moment. Now it was here. Of course she wanted to show him. They had shared everything else together, why not this? But she was terribly scared, too, scared of his reaction.

"I'm going to close my eyes," she said finally, "and turn around. I'm not sure I want to see the expression on your face." But when she turned around—she was totally naked by this point—she did not close her eyes. What the hell, she thought, and she showed him everything, struggling to keep her hands at her sides. In truth, her curiosity had gotten the better of her: she just had to *know* what his real reaction would be. His face would give away his true feeling instantly.

John studied her for a long moment. "It doesn't look bad at all," he said in a matter-of-fact voice that just couldn't have been faked. The straight line of the incision went down her chest, but she didn't have the bumps and indentations or hideous cross-hatching often associated with major surgery. "Strong did a nice job," he said almost begrudgingly.

Christine was surprised and relieved by his attitude: he really didn't care about it, it didn't seem to repulse him. They were still together. She threw herself at him, hugging him tightly.

"Because of the way he made the incision I'll still have some cleavage when I wear my 'falsie,' " she said. "It's amazing. When I get reconstructed in six months, you'll hardly know anything happened at all."

"I love you," John said. "I don't care about anything as unimportant as this."

He eased her down onto the bed and began to kiss her all over. At first she felt uncomfortable, still uneasy. Her mind was spinning with the complexities of the past month, and she was afraid to let go of a single one of her problems. Soon, very soon, however, the champagne and the strength of their love took over, and all the dross seemed terribly unimportant. The only thing that mattered was John and his love for her—that was what life was all about. To have been rejected by him at that moment would have been the worst blow, far worse than the physical loss of a breast. For she really would have been alone then. But since she had him, what did anything else matter?

It was one of those moments of love that would always stand out in her mind, one of those she would think of when she thought back on her love life at its best, as something really special, almost mystical in its intensity. She didn't realize how much she had longed for him these past days, or how deeply she missed his presence when he was gone.

Afterward, they lay on the bed in the afterglow of their passion. They luxuriated in their feelings and in what was, for them, the almost decadent pleasure of afternoon lovemaking. Outside, the world of business went on its frenetic way: inside here, behind their shuttered windows, they had constructed a little world of their own, and for an hour or two, at least, nothing could touch them.

Christine lay next to John, with his body snuggled up against her protectively, the way they often did at night. My own bed, she thought, wriggling against the clean sheets, the joy of being in my own bed. It was something you appreciated only when you had been away from it.

Softly, she started crying, waking him up from his stupor.

"Wh—what's the matter?" he asked, startled. He had been anticipating problems and had been relieved—but still cautious —when Chris responded so well.

"I'm so happy," she sobbed.

"So you cry?"

"It's so wonderful, John. It's *too* much. This is one of the best moments of my life. Isn't that weird? I should be miserable, right? But you've made me so happy."

PART TWO
Spring

Mildred

Mildred's lump was growing larger. There was no avoiding it. Every time she undressed, it was the first thing she saw. She knew she would have to seek medical help soon. But first she must prepare Carol for the worst. It was typical of her to think first about her children and to want to spare them the pain and mental anguish, even though they were a lot stronger than she gave them credit for.

Her friend, Molly Kagan, had had a mastectomy for breast cancer some years before. She had undergone surgery, radiation, and chemotherapy and had survived. So Mildred invited Molly to have lunch with her and Carol at the Four Guys Diner in Flatlands. They talked briefly about her operation. It was good: Carol could see that Molly was a fully functioning human being, driving her car, shopping, eating out, despite what had happened to her.

Later, when they dropped Carol off at her house in Sheepshead Bay, Mildred and Molly sat in the car and talked.

"So what's up with you?" Molly asked. "You seem troubled."

"I'm fine. It's just . . . oh, what's the use. Molly, I'm worried. I found something. . . ."

"A lump?"

Mildred nodded. This was the first person she had told.
"When? When did you find it?"
"Well, it's been a while. In the winter."
"And you didn't tell anybody about it since then?"
Milly shook her head. "I would have gone to see my internist," she said lamely, "but you know he retired and moved down to Florida."
"And he's the only doctor in the phone book?" asked Molly angrily.
"I didn't want to go to a breast man. I knew what he would say. And besides, the kids." She shrugged; she knew her excuses sounded weak. But for her they were still rational, or at least had been at the time.
"Here's what you have to do. There's a doctor here in Brooklyn who treated me and a number of my friends. He's wonderful. He's a *mensch,* Mill, a real person. This guy will tell you the truth, whatever it is. His name is Leslie Elliott Strong."

Yet still Mildred did not act. It was weeks later that she got out the piece of paper on which Molly had written the breast doctor's name and finally made an appointment. The reason she finally called him was that something very peculiar had begun to happen: not only did she still have the lump, larger and more menacing than ever, but there was now an indentation in the skin—as if the point of the umbrella had made a permanent dent in her flesh.

Dr. Strong's office was on Prospect Park West, in one of the loveliest sections of Brooklyn. It was early spring, and the buds on the trees across the street were starting to open. The office also served as the Brooklyn headquarters of the Breast Health Program. Mildred, accompanied by her son and daughter, was early for her appointment. As they waited, Strong's nurse gave them copies of the *BHP Bulletin,* a newsletter Strong published every three months.

"Would you like to see the movie?" she asked them.
"Movies? What fun," said her son. They all laughed.
"I don't know how much fun it is," said Susan, "but you might find it informative. It's a film we made on the subject of breast self-examination." She put a cassette in a VCR, and the film came on a TV monitor in a corner of the office.

Other waiting patients turned their chairs to watch it as well.

A middle-aged, attractive woman stood naked to the waist in front of the camera, while the narrator began to recite the statistics of breast disease.

"Mmm, soft-core porn," said her son.

"Quiet," said Mildred seriously. "This is important stuff."

The woman sat in front of a mirror and examined her breasts for a long moment.

"Is there any inequality in the size of your breasts?" asked the narrator, a man. "This is usually normal, but you have to be on the lookout for any changes. Has one breast, for example, recently become lower than the other?"

Carol glanced over at her mother. She shook her head.

"Now look at the nipple area," said the voice. "Has one nipple become turned in? Is there a discharge? Squeeze the nipple very gently, but without bruising." The naked woman followed his instructions. "And remember to always look on the inside of your bra for any sign of a discharge."

Mildred's son was beginning to feel a bit uncomfortable, but the women—his sister included—seemed rapt with attention.

"Look at the skin of the breasts. Are there any changes? For instance, do you notice any puckering or dimpling? Is there a rash or a change in the texture of the skin? Lift up the breasts, if necessary, to look at the undersurface."

An overweight woman at the rear of the room laughed nervously.

"Now raise your hands above your head and study the upper part of the breast that leads into the armpit. Now is there any swelling or puckering of the skin?"

The woman on the screen did as she was told, with a somewhat blasé expression on her face.

"Next, lie down in a relaxed and comfortable position. Many women prefer to do this part of the examination in the bath. Examine your left breast with your right hand. Use the front part of the flat of your hand and keep your fingers straight and close together. The important thing is to modulate the pressure in your hand, for if you press too hard, your sensation will be dulled, and if you press too lightly, you won't be able to feel deeply enough. Practice makes perfect. Make sure you do not *pinch* the breast, because if you do, you may feel lumps even in normal breasts."

The woman rested her left arm under her head while she massaged her ample left breast. "Slide your hand over the breast now," said the voice, "starting at the armpit and moving across the breast above the nipple to the center, pressing to feel for any lumps. Now repeat the action, this time from the outside moving inward below the nipple.

"Now, finally slide your hand over the nipple, in order to be sure that you have felt all parts of the breast. Feel now for lumps along the top of the collarbone and in the armpit. When you have done this, and are sure you have covered the entire breast, you are done. That completes the examination of the left breast. Now, on to the right breast. . . ."

"It seems so simple," her son said. "Did you ever do this?"

"No," Mildred whispered.

"How come?"

"It's . . . scary," she said, shuddering. "I was afraid I might find something."

Susan came over to them. "Dr. Strong will see you in his office now, Mildred."

Mildred rose and asked her children to stay put: she would rather face this alone.

"What can I do for you?" Strong asked.

"Well, I have a peculiar problem," Mildred said. "I was hit by an umbrella some months ago and I have a little indentation where the umbrella poked me."

Strong looked at her a bit dubiously. Many patients associated the development of breast disease with a blow or bruise, although that was not the case.

Mildred looked at the pictures on the wall of the examining room. These depicted breast self-examination—the same thing she had just been shown by Strong's nurse in the videotape. There were also pictures of the early signs of breast cancer. Her heart froze when she saw one entitled "dimpling and skin retraction." It looked just like her breast.

When Strong had her lie down and began to feel her he immediately felt the tumor—it was hard and hot. What Mildred was calling "an indentation" of the skin was actually the textbook picture of one kind of carcinoma of the breast. Strong had her lie down, and he carefully felt under her arms, or what he called her "axilla." His heart sank: this very cheerful, lively woman, with her colorful jewelry and *Chai* ring, not only had cancer, but it had already spread to the lymph nodes and probably beyond. The nodes were already palpably enlarged, hard and immobile in the vicinity of the tumor.

He had her sit up. "I don't mean to be too personal," he said, "but are you still active sexually?"

"Yes, I am," said Mildred, a bit surprised by the question.

"Then how is it your husband hasn't felt this and made you come in sooner?"

"I've never let him feel there. I just don't want to tell him and make him worry."

It never failed to astound Strong. Here was a woman—youthful and attractive for her age, with a wonderful sense of humor and a keen intelligence in her eyes, who delayed coming to see a doctor for weeks and months after discovering the lump. And now her nodes were heavily involved—a small detail that in itself could mean her life.

He asked her to get dressed again.

"Is someone from your family here?" he asked, when she was seated again opposite him in the office.

The minute she heard that she knew.

"As a matter of fact, both my daughter and my son are outside," she said soberly. "But I'd rather you told me first. Don't worry, I can take it."

"I'm sorry to tell you this, Mildred," said Strong, "but all the indications are that you have breast cancer, mammary carcinoma. The news is not good. Let me explain.

"In the Breast Health Program we like to offer surgical alternatives for the treatment of breast cancer. Unfortunately, these alternatives are not available to you, Mildred, because of the advanced condition of your tumor—what we call stage three cancer. The lymph nodes are involved and the tumor is over five centimeters, almost the size of a walnut.

"The only way we can now get local control is by a modified radical mastectomy. This involves removal of the breast and the lymph nodes under the arm, but with preservation of all the muscles of the chest wall. Because the tumor is in the center of the breast and the axillary, or armpit, lymph nodes are involved, it is also highly likely that the lymph nodes in the internal mammary chain"—he drew a line with his finger down his own breastbone— "are also involved. This means that you will also have to have a post-operative course of radiation therapy. The radiation will be delivered to the breast area itself, as well as the neck, or supraclavicular area, and the chest wall, so that the ribs do not become involved.

"Finally, you will have to have chemotherapy. There is a good chance that this tumor has spread throughout the body if it has spread as far as the lymph nodes. To deal with this systemic aspect of the disease you will need a year of chemotherapy. I will make an appointment for you to see Dr. Vogel."

Mildred was stunned, but deep in her heart, she wasn't really surprised. In a sense, she had known the worst somehow from the time she first spotted the growth months before. Everything since then—her theories about the umbrella, her hopes that it was benign, or that it would be controlled with what Molly had called a tiny lumpectomy—were simply delaying tactics, self-delusions.

In a way she felt terribly ashamed of herself. All her life she had prided herself on her practicality, her levelheadedness, and her strength, and now . . . suddenly, all her frustration and anger with herself turned into anger toward the doctor.

"How the hell can you say such a thing?" she yelled. "How can you *tell*, when you haven't even taken a mammogram or a biopsy or anything?" These damn doctors, she thought. And it was right what they said: surgeons were the worst. Why had she listened to Molly? And why did her damn internist have to move to Florida anyway? He would have told her the truth, or at least he wouldn't have been so eager to cut her open.

"Listen, dear," said Strong, frustrated but still patient. "You can rest assured that a mammogram will be taken of your breasts before the operation. We follow thorough procedures. First of all, instruction in breast self-examination, such as you received this afternoon. Then, the physical examination. This will be followed by pre-operative mammograms. We do this to learn more about the tumor, to see if there is any pathology in the opposite breast, and to establish a baseline, to see if there are any changes taking place in that breast over time. After the biopsy you will get a chance to go home and then come back for a discussion, in which all options will be discussed."

He could tell, however, that she was not concentrating on what he was telling her. He tried so hard to make the topic rational and comprehensible, yet often emotions got in the way. It wasn't difficult to see why, either.

"If you don't mind, Mildred," Strong said, "I'd like to get your family in here." She became calmer as soon as her son and daughter were by her side.

"I understand how upsetting this must be," said Strong. "The best thing for you to do in this situation is to get a second opinion. In fact, it is the policy of the Breast Health Program to provide a list of names of other breast surgeons in the New York area so that you make a meaningful comparison. Or you can go to a doctor of your own choosing, if you prefer. The important thing is that you do go, Mildred, and don't put this off again, the way you did before."

"But how can you tell this is cancer?" Carol asked. She had started crying as soon as she heard the diagnosis, while her mother remained dry-eyed.

"If I can't recognize this I'd better give up practice," Strong said emphatically. On a prescription paper Strong wrote out for her what he thought needed to be done:

> *Modified Radical Mastectomy:*
> 1) Breast
> 2) Lymph glands of the armpit
> 3) No chest wall muscles are to be removed
> *If the lymph glands are positive:*
> Then you will need
> Chemotherapy.

Millie put the wallet away in her black alligator bag. The three of them, mother, daughter, and son, stood outside the door of the office. It was getting dark out. Finally her son broke the silence and said, "A nice guy in a lousy job."

For her second opinion, Mildred chose the doctor who had operated on her for a benign thyroid tumor some years before. By coincidence, he happened to know Leslie Strong.

His own diagnosis was exactly the same as Strong's, almost down to the very words.

"Listen, Mildred," he said gravely. "I worked with Leslie Strong for four years at Downstate when he was there. If he says it's cancer, you can believe that it is."

"You sound like the Bobbsey Twins," she said, and went off looking for a third opinion.

She went to the doctor who had performed a partial hysterectomy on her long ago. She only had to look at his face as he examined her and she knew.

"What are you wasting your time and your money for?" he asked angrily. "Everyone is going to tell you the same thing."

She felt trapped. Surgery. Radiation. Chemotherapy. It was unthinkable. Yet it was real. But why bother? If she was going to die, she might as well die with some dignity, and without all the pain and inconvenience that modern medicine seems to specialize in. She had never been a medicine person, had always sought to live sanely and simply and to believe in nature's healing powers.

Her friend Molly, however, was persuasive: "Do you think I'd be alive today if it hadn't been for treatment? Untreated cancer is fatal. Period. At the very least, if you get treatment, it will prolong your life. Don't you owe that to your children and to Phil?"

The appeal to her motherly instincts was an unbeatable argument, and Molly was shrewd enough to know that.

And so, a week later, she was back with Dr. Strong, who scheduled surgery for her at Methodist for the following Tuesday.

"Well, you don't have to give up your practice," she said, laughing—more at herself than anyone. "I'm sorry if I called you names the other day. You didn't deserve it. But I still wonder if you're not in some kind of collusion with your Bobbsey Twin over there."

"I'm glad to see you've kept your sense of humor," said Leslie. She was like a different person from the one who had exploded at him in the office.

"Honey, if you've lost your sense of humor, you've lost everything. Laughter is the greatest medicine of all. And to prove there are no hard feelings, I brought you a present."

She handed him a box and he opened it, blushing slightly. Inside were half a pound of nut-filled, buttery *ruggaluch*, the kind that are only produced right by obscure bakeries in the far reaches of Brooklyn.

"Mmm," he said, holding one up to his nose. "Not so great for the diet! But still, the nicest present I've received all year."

Monday at noon Mildred Rosenbloom was at the admitting office of Methodist Hospital. Her son and her daughter were with her: she asked Phil not to come because she knew how much hospitals upset him. When the man with the wheelchair came, she said to them, "What's the sense of hanging out here —go do whatever you want to do. You can come back and visit me tonight."

They looked at each other. Carol was afraid to let her go. In her mind, somewhere, was the thought that her mother would disappear from her, be whisked out of her life. She had a friend at the Head Start program whose father had had a heart attack. It was not supposed to be serious and her father urged her to go out and get herself something to eat. When she came back, however, the bed was empty. In that short time he had had another attack and had died. The story had always stayed with her, although she had not known the man. She desperately feared the same thing would happen to her mother, although she knew this was not the kind of illness where things happen so suddenly and dramatically.

"Go, go, go," Mildred said with mock impatience. "You're making me nervous, both of you."

"Do you have everything, Mom?" asked her son a bit dubiously.

"Everything but my 'bobby,'" she said. Her "bobby" was a family joke, a pet pillow that went everywhere with her.

"You didn't bring it?" asked her daughter, concerned. "Want me to bring it back for you?"

Mildred rolled her eyes up. "Are you kidding? At my age they'd kick me out of the hospital altogether," she said. "Now get out of here. I'll see you tonight." She thought for a moment. "Bring your father back with you," she added as she waved good-bye.

Mildred quickly made herself at home in the hospital. Her roommate was another of Dr. Strong's patients, Nancy Browne.

"What have they got you in here for?" Mildred asked. She had a strong sense of curiosity.

"Breast," Nancy practically whispered. "Tumor."

Oh my God, thought Mildred. It's one thing to go through this when you're my age, when you've got a forty year–plus relationship with a wonderful guy like Phil. He had been so wonderful about it, too. What was that he had said? "What do I care? So I'll love the other breast twice as much." That was beautiful. It brought tears to her eyes just thinking about it. But a girl like this!

"How old are you, darling?"

"Twenty-six," said the girl.

"A tumor?"

The girl struggled to remember the medical terminology. "They gave it a name. I can't remember. But they think it's going to be all right." She sounded as if *she* wasn't as sure as *they*.

"You know what you have to do? Have them write it all down for you." Mildred reached into her bag, pulled out her well-worn purse, and unfolded a small piece of paper. It was the sheet of Dr. Strong's prescription pad with his diagnosis written on it. "This I keep with me all the time. I'll keep this always," she said proudly.

The young woman studied the sheet. "You're having a mastectomy?" she asked, in awe.

Mildred nodded. "Probably. I'm going in for my biopsy now, but they're pretty sure I'll need a mastectomy."

"How do you keep so . . . cheerful?"

"You have to," said Mildred. "It's the only way to survive."

"True," said the girl. "But I'm so afraid . . . of all this."

"Well, my heart goes out to you," said Mildred. "Are you married?"

The girl shook her head. "I have a boyfriend, but he's in the army right now."

"Well, you'll be okay. I have a feeling. Don't you remember what Dr. Strong told you? Four out of five of these breast lumps turn out to be benign. You know what that means? Eighty percent are not cancer. Only twenty percent are cancer, and that's mainly in women my age or older. In fact, they say that breast cancer only begins to become a really major problem in the thirty- and forty-year-old age group. But in the young—like you —or the old it's not as big a deal."

"Is that true?" Nancy said. "Four out of five are nothing?"

"Why, in your case," said Mildred, warming to her role as counselor, "it's probably more like nine out of ten. That's pretty good odds."

They sat speaking like this for a while, but Mildred couldn't keep still. She was a doer and she wanted to help out.

"Look," she said to the nurse finally, "I'm sick of just waiting around here. Give me something to do. I'm a pretty good psychiatrist. Want me to go around and talk to some of your depressed patients? Cheer them up?" The head nurse laughed. "Okay, then, how about filing? Can I do some filing for you?"

"Here, Mrs. Rosenbloom," one of the nurses said, laughing. "Why don't you get to work on these? We need these bottles put back in the case. Do you think you can do that?"

Already it was known that there was a "character" on the floor. Into the boring routine of Methodist 5 had come a live wire. Each of the nurses on both the outgoing and oncoming shifts had made a point to come by the desk to chat with her, and each of them was quickly on a first-name basis with Mildred.

In the midst of all this activity, Dr. Strong arrived, amazed to see his patient not in bed, but sitting at the desk doing manual labor.

"Well, I see you haven't been wasting any time getting to know people," said Strong. "But what are you going to do for an encore?"

Mildred laughed: it was like a big party. "Well, I've been saving that for you, Dr. Strong." She reached into her plastic shopping bag. "This is something special. I know you've had a hard day and you're probably tired and hungry."

Out came a stained paper bag and in it were four delicious potato knishes.

"The best thing for an afternoon pick-me-up," she said, breaking the salted knishes into pieces and handing them around to the outstretched hands of the hospital workers.

Dr. Strong

It had taken over a year of steady work, but the Breast Health Program of New York had become a reality. Strong, with Dorothy Wayner's help, had drawn up a 10-Point Early Detection Annual Program as well as a Statement of Goals (see Appendix). The essence of this was summed up in the slogan of the BHP: Education, Diagnostics, and Treatment Alternatives for all Breast Disease.

Women who enrolled in the BHP—and at first these were entirely made up of Strong's Brooklyn and Manhattan practices—received two breast examinations a year; individual training by Strong himself in breast self-examination; a complete physical examination and a complete updated medical history; a diagnostic work-up, including mammogram, thermogram, and needle aspiration, as well as educational programs, including the newsletter that was being readied for the press.

The first problem Strong confronted was to get other doctors to join the program. He was dealing with physicians who, like himself, were in private practice. Although they were all affiliated in one way or another with major hospitals, they had chosen to go into practice for themselves rather than work as salaried employees for hospitals, corporations, or research centers. This was an important distinction. As a rule, these were very independent-minded people, often more ambitious and self-willed than their colleagues in large institutions. On the other hand, the medical profession being what it is, they were fearful of doing anything that would offend their peers, who served as their sources of referral.

It took some hard convincing on Strong's part to get some of them to join. To assuage their concerns, Strong agreed to submit his Breast Health Program *Bulletin* to them all beforehand. If he didn't get any negative reaction, he would assume he was free to publish the articles.

Others saw the need for the BHP immediately and endorsed it quickly. Some were simply disgusted with the inadequate education women were receiving about their breast problems and saw this as a way to help. To some, it also served as a valuable source of patient referrals.

By the end of the first year, Strong had assembled an impressive letterhead, with thirty-three professionals on it, in such disciplines as radiology, obstetrics and gynecology, plastic surgery, oncology, internal medicine, and radiotherapy. A psychotherapist, Dr. Gerald Lucas, was even persuaded to join.

Most of these specialists were within walking distance of one or another of Strong's offices, so that patients could be served easily. All of them were board-certified in their fields, and had impressive records in dealing with breast cancer and other breast diseases. And all of them were the kind of doctor Strong himself would want if *he* had a serious medical problem.

The problem now was to "sell" the BHP to some of the large institutions of New York as a way of finding and treating breast cancer in their employees and members. The concept of early detection was not new—it stemmed from the idea that the sooner a cancer is discovered the greater the chance of survival. But no one had aggressively gone out and incorporated this concept into an actual program for saving lives. Strong soon discovered why.

They met in the board room of a large multinational oil corporation on Sixth Avenue. Strong and Dorothy Wayner were there, of course, and around the table sat the medical directors, personnel managers, or administrators of ten large corporations.

Strong made his presentation, which he had rehearsed with

Dorothy the night before. He emphasized the statistics, so frightening and impressive: 112,000 new cases a year of breast cancer in the United States alone, with the incidence rising year by year.

One million breast biopsies a year.

One in twelve women developing breast cancer some time in her life.

Twenty-five to fifty percent of all American women developing fibrocystic disease, or "lumpy breasts."

He showed them the article he xeroxed from a magazine on the major causes of death. In the 35–44 age group *the* major cause of death among all women was breast cancer, and it continued in the top three until a woman reached her seventies. "We want to change these abominable statistics," Strong emphasized. The executives assembled around the smooth wooden table seemed attentive and impressed by his facts and figures.

Then Strong outlined his plans for the Breast Health Plan. He showed how, through early detection, good treatment, and preventive care, hundreds of lives could be prolonged or saved in their institutions. He explained who his consultants were, and about their qualifications. After an hour, he summed up with an appeal to them to join the program.

"What you're talking about sounds good, Dr. Strong," said the head personnel officer for the transit system. "But you know what a financial crunch we're in. How can we afford such a program when we're cutting back older ones?"

Strong was ready for this tack.

"The cost of *not* treating breast disease is greater," he emphasized.

"A case that is detected early is much less expensive to treat, and the woman has more productive years ahead of her. Besides, all we're asking for is two thousand dollars from each of you. For that two thousand dollars, you can send us one hundred women of your choosing. We'll work on them based on any risk factors you choose—age, the presence of lumpy breasts, nationality. That works out to twenty dollars a patient, and for that they'll receive a complete examination of the breast.

"For individual patients in the program the cost is also very inexpensive. At the present time it costs forty-five dollars to join the program as an individual. For that they receive a complete diagnostic workup, and a mammogram with us, which costs an additional thirty-five dollars."

"That doesn't seem like a lot," said a young personnel manager from the telephone company. "I had one last month, and it cost me one hundred twenty-five dollars."

"Precisely," said Strong. "And so for eighty dollars they get complete breast care for a year. But for you we're willing to do that for just twenty dollars, just so that we can get you incorporated into our program."

"But don't adequate facilities exist already?" asked a middle-aged gentleman from a major electronic manufacturer. "I mean there are so many doctors, so many hospitals. What about the famous 'war on cancer'? What about the major cancer centers?"

"We feel our program is superior," said Strong confidently. "There's nothing wrong with the facilities at the major centers," said Strong. "But you have to realize that a big cancer center may have up to five thousand employees, including hundreds of different doctors. They have huge teaching operations. And so very often a woman will be seen by a doctor and then never see that person again. Patients can get lost in the shuffle. As in all big institutions there is a tendency toward red tape and bureaucracy. Policies are set and then they remain inflexible, despite the individual needs of the patient. And everyone is an individual, after all. The Breast Health Program is a confederation of specialists who deal with breasts. But each patient will be under my personal supervision, and will be dealing with people I know are both competent and concerned. Everyone knows what can go wrong at a major hospital when you become just another number."

Quite a few of the people nodded their heads in agreement: some had personal anecdotes and grievances they would have loved to pour out.

"What about the American Cancer Society?" asked an executive from a textile company. "Don't they do this? I give every year and now you're telling us they're inadequate."

"Well, first of all, I myself am affiliated with the ACS. I'm a member of the executive board of the Brooklyn Division of the Society, as well as a member of the professional education and grant committee. But the problem is that the ACS can only make recommendations; it cannot put those recommendations into effect. For instance, the ACS says that mammography is necessary for women at the age of thirty-five. But who actually takes responsibility for that woman's breasts?"

"The woman's own doctor, her gynecologist," said a medical director.

"Well, many women do not have a personal gynecologist. Some recent statistics I saw showed that half the people in the country have no personal physician at all. And many gynecologists do not do thorough breast examinations. That is not really their specialty." Strong thought of Ernestine Merryman, the case that had actually inspired the whole project.

"What exactly do you want from us, Strong?" asked the medical director of the oil company who was hosting the meeting.

"If you'll look in your folder, you'll see the Complete Program Summary." There was a shuffling of papers. "We're limiting the program to ten corporations. We're looking for a one-year commitment, as a minimum. Based on the incidence rate of cancer by age, the total population of women should be selected in various age categories, but the bulk of them in the thirty-five to forty-nine-year-old range, which is the most dangerous period. Each corporation will receive a detailed breakdown of data derived from the medical reports.

"I've spoken to you of the cost. But I think I can show you that this is very cost-effective. You see, based on the incidence of breast cancer, nine percent of the population (or a potential eighteen out of two hundred) may already be in need of surgical treatment for the breast. If the program, however, detects cancer in only four women at an early stage, thereby avoiding a modified mastectomy, hospitalization, and repeated treatments, the program effectively could save an estimated thirty thousand to thirty-five thousand dollars in medical costs.

"And this is not to mention the mental and emotional costs," Strong added, departing from his text. "The incalculable suffering of these women. The BHP is striving to raise women's awareness about new medical advances. It is a place in New York City where women are welcome to come and just talk . . . to question . . . to get answers about all their breast problems and health."

He was finished and felt emotionally drained. Somehow he wasn't getting the enthusiastic response he had anticipated, but he just didn't know why. Perhaps he had anticipated too much. Dorothy, however, secretly shot him a thumbs-up sign. There was polite applause.

The chairman broke the meeting for a buffet lunch, and people circulated. Everyone seemed friendly. After lunch, the corporate participants met for about fifteen minutes without Strong or Dorothy Wayner. When they came back in, the man from the host corporation tapped his pencil on his glass.

"We want to thank you, Dr. Strong, for giving us this opportunity to view your program. It is most impressive. We would like to join in." Strong looked over at Dorothy, who beamed at him. "However, we all use the major health diagnostic services, such as Life Extension Institute or Executive Health. We, therefore, all feel we'd be duplicating the services they already provide by joining up with you at this time. Also," he added, a bit less formally, "you know what the economy's like at the present. We have to cut the frills."

Strong almost screamed out in anger: don't you realize that women are going to die on account of you and your economics! Haven't I explained to you that you're going to save money in the long run? What the hell is wrong with you and your kind? At one time, perhaps, he would have yelled this. But he knew that word would quickly get around and that would be the end of the program. For the sake of the women, he would bite his tongue—although it didn't do much for his own mental health to have to suppress his rage.

"But don't worry, Dr. Strong," said the administrator of a publishing firm who had seemed sympathetic. "If we run into a major problem we'll be sure to call you."

Gladys

Her daughter Polly had insisted, and so Gladys Kalin had come to see Dr. Fine. It was ridiculous, really. She had lived with these damn varicose veins for thirty years. She was fifty-two years old, and could live with them for the rest of her life as well.

Gladys didn't like doctors or hospitals. Growing up on the East Side of New York, in the days of the Third Avenue "El," she had learned to avoid them at all costs. Who hadn't heard about the "black bottle," the mysterious poison they used to dispatch poor people at the old Bellevue Hospital? If they didn't do you in, at the very least they'd rob you blind. To put it mildly, Gladys Kalin wasn't overly impressed with the medical profession. And thank God she had remained healthy all these years. She intended to remain well—mainly by keeping away from all medical men.

But Polly was insistent and cleverly played on her vanity. Gladys was still quite attractive for fifty-plus. She didn't look particularly Irish—people sometimes even mistook her for Italian, with her dark bobbed hair and warm, chocolate-colored eyes. She was proud of her figure—a bit overweight, to be sure, but well-proportioned—and proud of her ample bust. In fact, the only thing that bothered her were these purplish varicose veins that had popped out on her legs after Polly was born. Her first husband hadn't minded, but he was long gone—succumbing finally to the complications of diabetes that had made their life a medical nightmare for twenty years. Her new husband, Sam, occasionally made cracks about them. That bothered her, even though he meant no harm, and so she decided she would at least talk to this Dr. Fine.

Dr. Barry Fine's office was in a professional building in Paramus, only about fifteen minutes from Gladys' suburban ranch house. He was a wiry man, about forty, in good shape, with tennis memorabilia on every wall.

"Do you still do the same kind of operation—the three stages?" She indicated the marks on her legs. She had heard about how extensive an operation it really was.

"Yes, we do," said Fine.

"Well, forget it then. I don't want to be cut up, thank you. I'll wear elastic stockings and get by. I've gotten by these fifty-two years; I think I'll survive."

Fine looked at her in amazement. There was something attractive about the woman—she was warm and spontaneous—but also something maddeningly frustrating. He felt like screaming: "Then what the hell are you doing here? Wasting my time?" but he knew that wouldn't do any good. Polly, who was his telephone-company sales representative, had pleaded with him to see her mother. But what for?

"At least, while you're here, let me give you a general checkup," he said, his breath hissing out in frustration. "Have you had one lately?"

"What, a checkup, you kidding?" said Gladys, in her abbreviated style of talking in which she often swallowed verbs, nouns, or adjectives helter-skelter.

"Okay? At least you'll get something for your money."

"Sure, why not?" she said. If she was dropping forty bucks for a consultation, she thought, she might as well get something for it.

She disrobed a bit reluctantly. Undressing in front of a man, even a white-clad doctor like this, was always something of an embarrassment. Her grandmother—God rest her soul—had brought her and her two sisters up as proper ladies, after their father and mother had both died young. Grandma was a character, the type you don't see anymore. She cursed and carried on, especially against the various nationalities that had the nerve to try and share New York City with the Irish. She drank two quarts of Rheingold a day and smoked a pipe until she died at ninety-six. But she raised them to be "proper ladies." When they went to dances, they had to cross their arms over their chests to hide their growing bosoms. If you showed any cleavage at all, you were a "hussy." Of course, times had changed, but some of those attitudes still clung to Gladys. She removed her brassiere reluctantly and let her breasts hang free. Dr. Fine took in the attractiveness of her breasts and the lady's ambiguous attitude in one knowledgeable glance. He knew the type. She probably never examined herself, either, or allowed others to examine her. He began feeling her breasts in methodical circles.

"Do you examine yourself regularly?" he asked as he kneaded.

"What, are you kidding?" she said, laughing.

"Why not?" he asked.

"I guess I leave that to my husband," said Gladys, laughing. But it rang false to both of them.

Fine went along, working systematically, and then he stopped and went back over the same area. He continued on, then came back to the same spot, as if puzzled by something.

The doctor stood up from his stool and walked to the other side of the room.

"I'm glad you let me examine you," he said, but his voice sounded different now. "There's a . . ." He searched for the proper words. ". . . strange irregularity in your left breast," he said.

"A what?" she exclaimed, perplexed.

"A strange irregularity," he repeated. "You're going to have to get looked at right away," he added.

"Looked at?" said Gladys.

"A mammogram," said the doctor. "An X ray of the breast."

Gladys thought about it for a moment. She had a friend, someone she knew from the Bronx hardware store where she worked, who went every year for a mammogram and a Pap test. She swore by them, and tried to get Gladys to go, saying they were painless and worthwhile. Gladys had never had either, but had always thought about getting one. Maybe this was the time.

"One of my colleagues over at Barnard Memorial can give it to you," said Fine. "Or you can use someone else. The choice is yours. But I strongly suggest that you do it right away."

Don't push me, thought Gladys. Push too hard and I'll just walk out of here. But then again, what the hell do I have to lose? I might as well get it done. But, win or lose, she thought, that's as far as it'll ever go.

After the X rays were taken at Barnard—and they were indeed quite painless—she called Fine's office to get the results. He wasn't in: it was a Jewish holiday, and he would be out for the rest of the week.

"Isn't there anyone there *working?*" she asked in annoyance, and finally managed to raise one of Fine's partners, a Dr. Billy, who said nonchalantly that he would look for the results on Fine's desk.

When he came back, she could sense the change of attitude, like a little current of electricity coming over the phone. "Mrs. Kalin, they found an irregularity in the left breast. A mass. Dr. Fine *strongly* suggests that you get a biopsy."

"A biopsy?" she said. She knew what that meant, more or less. She had had enough friends with cancer to know all about it, and she was determined that it would never happen to her.

"Yes, if it's benign, then you're done with it," said Dr. Billy soothingly.

"And if it's whatchamacallit, malignant?"

"If it's malignant," said Dr. Billy, "then . . . well, it depends on how big it is. The only way we can find out, though, is to go in and look."

"Does that mean with a needle?" she asked. A little needle in the breast to draw out some cells would be no picnic, but it was something she could live with.

"No, we strongly suggest an open operation," Billy said, and he sounded nervous. "An excisional biopsy."

Glady got up from the kitchen table and stirred the beef stew she was making for her husband. She absentmindedly wiped some brown sauce that had splattered onto her new daffodil wallpaper.

"Okay," she said slowly. "I'll let him know. Tell the doctor I thank him very much and I'll think about it."

She had learned how to get rid of people on the telephone from years of practice at the store. People who wanted things from her . . . blood, sweat, tears, and more often than not, money. After all, she was a native New Yorker, not a hayseed out-of-towner, born yesterday. She knew these surgeons. Everyone was wise to them. This Dr. Fine was crazy if he didn't realize she saw through him and his type.

"Are you going to do anything about it?" asked Dr. Billy, getting a bit agitated.

The first word out of her mouth was "no," but she quickly modified this to a "maybe." She was still shocked by the whole thing, shocked and amazed. Me sick? How dare they even suggest it? She was healthy!

"If I were you, I wouldn't wait too long," said Dr. Billy, and he reluctantly said good-bye.

It was some time later that Gladys' daughter, Polly, ran into an old friend at Gumbo's, a watering hole in Paramus. The old friend was Dr. Fine's nurse.

"Polly, how'd your mother make out?" asked the nurse casually.

"Oh, great. Everything was great." Her mother had mentioned that Fine had found a little change in her breast, but that it had turned out to be nothing. It was the same story she had given Sam and her sisters.

"What do you mean, great?" the nurse blurted out.

"Yeah, she told me everything was copasetic."

"Polly," the nurse said gravely, "your mother needs a biopsy. She has a growth."

She could see the shock in Polly's eyes. Polly in some ways was the opposite of her mother: she took everything medical with immediate alarm, saw disaster lurking around every corner. "Hey, I feel bad. I'm not supposed to tell you this. I'm not supposed to divulge patients' medical records, you understand."

"You're crazy," said Polly angrily. "My mother's fine. She told me so herself. Told me and told her husband and told everyone."

"I'm crazy?" said the nurse. "Okay, I'm crazy. But maybe you'd better call Dr. Fine and find out what's really going on."

The next evening, Polly was waiting in the sunken living room of her mother's house when Gladys came home from work. She was tottering a bit humorously on her high heels—she never had learned how to walk comfortably in them, although she wore them every business day.

"Well, well, well, to what do we owe the honor?" Gladys asked nervously.

"Ma," said Polly angrily, "why did you lie to me?"

Gladys was surprised. "What the hell are you talking about? Calling your own mother a liar and . . ."

"Cut the crap, Ma," said Polly, livid now. "I spoke to Dr. Fine today. Called him up. He told me that you were supposed to have a biopsy for a lump in the breast. They *told* you that, but you never went."

"That's right," said Gladys.

"And can you tell me why?" said Polly, trying now to moderate her tone. She followed her mother into the TV room and positioned herself opposite her on the couch.

"Because . . . well, it's hard to explain. I don't know. I don't trust these doctors. They're all out for themselves. And, well, maybe I thought it would go away. You know," she said, laughing, "like the young girls who get pregnant and think, well, maybe it'll go away. Don't look, don't look, it's not there. If I'm quiet about it, nobody'll notice." The words shot out of her in her usual slapdash, rapid-fire way.

"Did it?" asked her daughter, knowing the answer.

"No," said Gladys, her eyes more watery than usual. "I check. It's still there."

"Have you told Sam about this?" Polly asked.

"You kidding?" she said. "You think he wants to hear this?"

"Ma, you'd better get your ass in gear. You've got to get to a hospital for that biopsy. I'll go with you."

"Yeah, well, maybe, we'll see." She zapped the TV with the remote control and the twenty-four-inch screen was suddenly filled with Dan Rather's face. She did a quick flip through the stations, and wound up with a *M*A*S*H* rerun. Klinger was giving away his dresses for the umpteenth time. End of argument.

"Ma," Polly yelled over the noise of helicopters and loudspeakers.

"Yeah, we'll see, we'll see," said Gladys, and she settled into the couch for her evening's entertainment.

A few days later there was a pink slip in Gladys' mailbox: a registered letter was at the post office waiting for her. All official things like that alarmed her. She went to the post office first thing in the morning, before work.

It was a letter from Dr. Fine, neatly typed, on good bond stationery. The language was technical and very formal. Fine was making a big thing about her lump, insisting that it was his duty to inform her that she *had* to get a biopsy. He insisted that she do something about her "irregularity." Don't procrastinate, he said, and all that garbage. At the end he said it didn't matter if she used him—he was a general surgeon—or somebody else, as long as she did *something*. Well, that was nice of him, she thought. At least he's not a money-grubber. Along with the letter was the radiologist's report describing the irregularity they had seen on the mammogram. Suspicion of CA, it said. Gladys took Fine's letter, folded it neatly, and tucked it away in her leather handbag.

Gladys had a friend, Maureen McConnell, whose husband had been diagnosed as having colon cancer. The doctors in New Jersey had given him three months to live. And so he had bought himself a plot and a stone, and invited all his friends—and enemies—to a farewell party. He thanked his friends for their help throughout the years and—everyone being fairly smashed—told off each and every enemy for what they had done to him, as long as twenty years before. They had a grand old time. It was a great way to go. The only trouble was, someone convinced him to get a second opinion at a big cancer center in New York City, and there the doctors did not agree with the first diagnosis. They shrank the tumor by radiation, and then removed it. A full year later the man held another huge party—this one a "recovery party." He invited the same people back and apologized to them.

So Gladys confided in Maureen McConnell, who told her, "Look, maybe it's nothing. Look at Joe, he was supposed to die in three months and now look at him. He's practically all better. The thing for you to do is to go to the top, go to New York, and find out what's really wrong with you. Chances are, it's nothing, but if it's something, you might as well go to the top. They'll fix you up in no time."

Gladys therefore went to the New York cancer center. With its hundreds of beds and state-of-the-art equipment, it would rank as a major hospital anywhere, and it dealt exclusively with cancer and allied diseases. She made an appointment to be seen by doctors in their Breast Clinic.

She sat in the huge, plushly furnished waiting room and waited. And waited and waited. By some administrative slipup, they had failed to put her name on the list. The longer she waited, the more upset she became. This center tended to attract not only the wealthiest but also the most serious cases of malignancy. Sitting there for four hours, Gladys felt like she was going to die. She had brought a book with her, but she could only stare in rapt fascination at the parade of sick people who traipsed before her on their way to therapy.

Imagine the in-patients, she thought, if these are the walking ones! There were people who looked like skeletons, like concentration camp victims. They had no color, or were a pale and sickly green. They staggered along with kidney-shaped vomit dishes held before them. Little kids, like Martians with dangly limbs. People with parts of their bodies missing. A man with a hole where his nose used to be. Incredibly, he lit up a cigarette as soon as he got outside! People with no hair, with hollowed-out parts showing. An incredible array of deformed, mangled, sad, and terribly resigned individuals. She couldn't tell where the ravages of nature left off and the ravages of medicine began. And I'm worried about myself, she thought . . . just look at these people! Whatever consolation lay in that thought vanished when she thought, Gee, if things got really bad would *I* look like that, too? At one point she wiped tears from her eyes for a little kid so fragile-looking that she thought he might break, shatter into a thousand pieces if someone so much as bumped into him. So this was what they meant by cancer treatment! No, thank you!

Finally, after four hours of this internal torment, she was called to the desk and asked whom she was waiting for. They had no record of her appointment. Gladys angrily announced she was going home. The lady behind the desk was terribly upset and personally took her upstairs.

Dr. Lisante, a breast surgeon, examined the X rays she had brought from New Jersey. As often happened, the doctors at the cancer center were unimpressed with the techniques practiced in the hinterlands, and he sent her down for a fresh set of mammograms. He called over another couple of doctors—one of them a young resident of some sort—and she overheard them discussing her case. It didn't sound good.

Dr. Lisante then examined her again.

He was a tall, thin man in his early fifties, with a pencil-line mustache.

"We can get you in next Monday," said Lisante curtly. "Be here before noon. You come in at the main entrance and turn immediately to your right for admittance. Once you're admitted, I'll come and see you."

He handed her two pieces of paper. One was a release to do a biopsy. The other, to her utter amazement, was a similar permission slip—only this one to do a mastectomy, to remove her breast!

"Whoa," she said, standing up. "Wait a minute. Don't push me, doctor. Why can't you just do one operation and then let me think about the other one?"

She had obviously hit a raw nerve, for the doctor stiffened and became even more distant. "We don't do things that way."

"Why can't you just wake me up and tell me what happened?" she shot back, "and then give me a chance to make my own decision. Make up my own mind. Don't push me into something that I may not have to do," she said, her eyes flashing with a strength the doctor had hardly expected. "I mean, you know all the ropes. I'm new at this. Don't rush me."

Lisante repeated, this time with visible anger, "We don't do things that way, Mrs. Kalin. The policy of the hospital is that you have to sign twice so we can have only one operation if the lump turns out to be malignant. I don't want you to blame me for charging you twice, once for each operation."

"But that's my choice," said Gladys, amazed at his obstinacy and at what was apparently the hospital's policy. She was trying to regain her composure, to find the right question to ask. There were so many on her mind.

"And what if I don't do anything? How long, in your professional opinion, do you think it would take before my body malfunctioned or the tumor spread?"

The doctor was clearly tired of these ignorant people who insisted on mishandling their own cases. "I have no crystal ball," he said angrily. "I have no time for such nonsense!" He stood up and walked out of the room.

Gladys was livid and completely lost control of herself. She yelled at his disappearing back, "You bastard! They never should have let you out of medical school!"

Then she broke down and cried bitterly. Lisante's nurse came into the room and thought Gladys was crying because of bad news. "Dr. Lisante says we've got a shortage of beds, but he's made an appointment for you for next Monday."

"No, it'll have to wait a while," said Gladys ironically. "Give the bed to someone else right now. I don't think I'm going to need it."

Martha

In the noisy neighborhoods of Brooklyn, you cherish the quiet moments. There are so few. Car alarms, box radios, neighbors' late-night TVs—one ends, the other begins. Then, suddenly, unexpectedly, the noise seems to stop. No truck on the way to a construction site, no motorcyclist burning rubber as he accelerates toward Long Island. Just silence. Your jaw relaxes a bit, you crane your neck around experimentally. You remember how it was when you were a child, when the world was so much quieter . . . and pleasanter.

Martha Bunim and her husband Ralph sat in the living room of their apartment in Brooklyn's Sheepshead Bay, enjoying the silence. It was a Monday afternoon in spring. Their daughter Melissa was away at college, in her freshman year. Their son Benjamin, or "B.J.," as he now preferred to be called, was at his experimental high school in Manhattan.

Martha sat with the guitar in her lap. She was playing Purcell, tunes from the *Fairy Queen*. Seventeenth-century stuff, before Bach. It anticipated the complexity of the German contrapuntal school, but had a certain sweetness and airiness all its own. Ralph raised his hand when she finished the "Dance of the Fairies."

"Something wrong?" she asked. She was sure she was no

good, that it was impossible to begin the guitar again at age forty and be any good.

"No, it's fine. Terrific," he said reassuringly—and it was true. She played very well indeed, and got better all the time. "It's just so *quiet* out there. Listen."

She laid the guitar down and cocked an ear. It had, indeed, grown quiet. "Country living again," she said, and they laughed. It was a private joke, something an old woman had said to them during the New York City blackout of 1965, just before their daughter was born. A household joke, one of the score of well-worn sayings that husband and wife passed back and forth as small change.

Just then a bus came churning around the corner and settled underneath their terrace window. They were half a block from the bus stop, but sometimes the bus drivers decided to wait there, their engines spewing fumes into the apartment, for reasons of their own. Martha and Ralph raised their eyebrows—each face a mirror of the other—and laughed.

"Too good to be true," said Ralph.

"What time is it?"

"Four," said Ralph. "I'd better get dinner started." He cooked all the meals and had been doing so for years, ever since he had left public relations and taken the risky step of being a free-lance science writer.

"What are we having?" she asked.

"Chicken cutlets, but don't ask for parmigiana, 'cause that's not on your diet."

"Great," she said ironically. "Damn, I haven't practiced enough and I have a lesson tomorrow. Do I have fifteen more minutes?"

"What else do you have to do?"

"I'd better take a shower. I don't want to rush. I like to rest up a little before I go to work."

Martha worked nights—the 7 P.M. to 3 A.M. shift in a type shop in the city. She was a skilled electronic phototypesetter. It was detailed, skilled, and exacting work. She enjoyed her job, but it was grueling and left little time for anything else. Thus, it had been a big step when she had decided to take up the guitar again after a six-year absence.

"Don't let me stay in the bath too long," she yelled, stripping off her clothes. Her body, at forty, was still youthful, a bit heavier than when they had started dating in high school twenty-five years before, but still lovely. Her breasts in particular were youthful, upturned and shaped like Venus de Milo's. She hurried down the hallway crowded with filing cabinets and excess book shelves.

Martha drew the bath and sat on the edge of the tub reading *Ovation* magazine, which had just arrived. She would soak for half an hour or so and then follow this up with a vigorous shower, while her husband prepared a delicious and dietetic dinner. Not a bad life, she mused, a faint smile on her face.

Ralph was into the vegetables, peeling the celery root to make a French-style crudité, when he heard the scream.

There were screams and screams. Like most of their overcrowded neighbors, they were a noisy family. But this was different. It was an emergency sound—a red light flashing. Panic. It sounded like something he had heard as a freshman in college when a kid thrust a frostbitten hand under the hot water faucet.

His shirttails flying, he tore into the living room, backtracked, and held onto the doorjambs of the bathroom, panting. There was Martha, standing up in a foot of water in the tub. She had cut the water and pulled back the curtain. What he noticed first was her color—she was ashen white and her black hair, lying in strings on her neck and shoulders, made her look even more ghostlike. She had grabbed a small beige towel and was holding it to her and her teeth were chattering. He expected to see blood, perhaps the kind of wound so deep that it takes seconds or minutes to come to the surface. But there was no blood.

He looked at her and then his heart sank from her expression, although he still hadn't grasped the nature of the terror in her eyes.

"What is it? What's wrong?" he screamed, almost angrily.

"I fe-f-felt something," she said, shuddering. He noticed for the first time that both her hands were clasped defensively over her left breast.

"What do you mean?" he asked, approaching a bit closer. The floor was wet, and he, quite absurdly, didn't want to dirty the tiles with his shoes.

"I felt something," she repeated. "Something in my breast."

He smiled nervously. She was an alarmist. Undoubtedly this was nothing, another false alarm. But something in her manner scared him.

He grabbed his big brown towel and said, "Come here." Unsteadily she lifted one foot, then the other, from the bath, and allowed him to drape the towel around her shoulders.

Ralph suddenly felt squeamish, almost light-headed. He had written a great deal about medicine, but the idea of some sort of uncontrolled growth in her body made him queasy.

"Let me feel," he said finally. He was trying to be tender, but his voice came out businesslike. Martha slowly peeled her hands from the breast and let him touch her. It was incredible. Imbedded in the upper outside part of her left breast was a lump. But that word hardly conveyed what he felt. It was something surprisingly large. It was an angular protrusion and had an out-of-place quality to it: it simply didn't belong; yet it was there.

"Does it hurt?" he asked gently.

"No, not at all."

For reasons he couldn't fathom he wished it did, wished it were sore and tender. That would be within the realm of ordinary experience. A cut, a bruise. Kiss it and make it better. This, however, was something strange, something that had just snuck up on them while they weren't looking.

Ralph felt a bit light-headed. The soap had slipped into the drain of the tub, where she had dropped it, and, almost in a trance, he watched its substance slowly oozing down the drain. He steadied himself. For one wild moment he felt like fleeing, letting her deal with it. But the moment passed.

"Come on, I'll help you get dressed." Sopping wet, she left her footprints on the floor of the hallway and then lay down on the bed.

"What the hell is it?" he asked. "Where did it come from? You had an examination before we went to Europe, right?"

She nodded, her face still pale.

"I think so," she said. "Both the Kurzes. He gave me a general exam, and I'm pretty sure he checked my breasts. And she gave me an internal exam. Yes, I remember her feeling my breasts." The Kurzes, Larry and Yang-nim, were their physicians, a husband-and-wife team of internist and gynecologist.

"Well, you've had lumps before," he said feebly.

"Nothing like this. I've always had lumpy breasts, but that comes and goes with my period. It runs in my family," she said. "This is different. It's, I don't know, harder. And rounder. And it doesn't hurt. My period lumps are usually quite sore."

He reached over and felt it again, a bit more confidently than last time, but still with a sort of awe. He could move it around with his fingers. It was like the pit of a mango, he thought. He stared at the breast. Was he imagining it, or could he see it pushing its way through the skin? Yes, definitely! The breast looked swollen, a bit misshapen at that point. He couldn't believe this was happening, but it was. Half an hour before, they had been sitting around, listening to music, their biggest immediate problem what to have for dinner. Suddenly they were fighting for her life, for their lives. For they had been together for most of their lives—they could hardly remember when they *weren't* together.

"You know," he said slowly, "if it really *wasn't* there when the Kurzes examined it . . ."

"It's growing very fast, isn't it?" she answered.

They had forgotten to put on the light and the blue-gray twilight filtered into the room, diffused off the water of Sheepshead Bay across the street. They sat for a moment like this, him stroking her cold hand.

"How did you find it?" he asked. "Tell me exactly what happened."

She told the classic story: she was soaping herself up and suddenly it was there. He remembered that breast self-examination classes usually taught women to soap themselves up in order to find lumps.

"It's like *it* came looking for *me*, honey," Martha said.

"What are we going to do?" he asked.

She shook her head. "Listen," she said slowly, "if I do have cancer . . ."

"What the hell are you talking about?" he screamed. He didn't want to hear it, wouldn't allow it. It was not cancer, not that. No, he wouldn't let it be.

"But if it is, I want—"

"Shut up," he said angrily, and she started to cry. He felt terrible, but not as terrible as if he had let her start speculating about her death, her funeral.

"Listen, this is nothing," he said, kissing her. "I'm sorry," he mumbled. "But I can't *stand* for you to talk that way, do you understand? Can't stand it. Nothing terrible is going to happen to you. Don't worry."

If only he believed that.

The Kurzes' office was in Park Slope, a lovely brownstone they had renovated into a combination office and residence.

Larry Kurz took her right in. Ralph sat in the dimly lit waiting room. They had been lucky. The Kurzes were in that afternoon and had an opening, or at least made one when they heard what the problem was.

"Well, you still have lovely breasts," he said as Martha disrobed.

She felt reassured by his warmth. "That's what people always said."

"Oh, you've heard that before?"

"Always," she said. "At least when I was younger."

"Well, let's see what the problem is here."

He made her lie down and he started to palpate her breasts. "Is this it?" he asked.

She nodded.

"Does this hurt?" he asked. She shook her head. He continued to probe and poke.

She had closed her eyes. When she looked up, the smile was gone. He seemed nervous and upset.

"I want Yang-nim to look at this," he said. He hurried out. A minute later Yang-nim, who always seemed a bit calmer than her husband, came into the room.

"Hi," she said. The tone was just right, friendly yet assured. "Let's have a look at you."

She felt again, her touch strong. Now the breast was growing tender, from all the poking and pulling, and Martha winced.

"Hurt?" Yang-nim said, surprised.

"Just sore."

She stood back. Larry stood back. They looked directly at each other.

"What is it?" asked Martha.

Yang-nim cleared her throat. "We want you to see a surgeon," she said.

"A surgeon?" Martha said. Her voice came out in a kind of screechy noise. "Why? What's wrong?"

"Don't be alarmed, dear," said Yang-nim. But she herself looked a bit alarmed. "The chances are good, no, *great*, that this is a benign growth. But we are not breast specialists. We want you to go to someone who is, who can really find out for you and take care of the problem."

"Then it's not cancer?" she asked.

"Yang-nim didn't say that," said Larry cautiously. "But to me it doesn't feel like a typical malignant lesion. Do you have a surgeon you want to use?"

Martha thought for a moment. The only surgeon she knew was the bastard who had botched her daughter's appendectomy a few years before. Besides, she wasn't sure she even *wanted* to see a surgeon.

"We know a person," said Yang-nim. "He practices in both Manhattan and Brooklyn. His name is Dr. Leslie Strong."

"Is he good?"

"Yes, he is," said Larry. "He started something called the Breast Health Program sometime back. It's a very interesting concept: an attempt to offer education, diagnostics, and treatment alternatives for all breast diseases. We think it's really a big advance on the management of breast problems. In fact, we're on the advisory board."

"All right. Give me the number then," said Martha.

"No, I think we'd better call him first," said Larry. "Will you be home? He'll call you tonight."

"No, but my husband will be home. He can ask the questions. I have to go to work."

Thinking about it later, a thousand thoughts ran around in her head. The strangest one had to do with the doctor's call. She had never heard of a doctor calling his patient before. Usually the patient had to make the first move. Did this mean that her condition was particularly serious? Did the Kurzes have something to say to Strong that they couldn't say to her, some secret information about her disease that they weren't telling her?

Well, that's the way doctors are, she thought. Cliquish. But they would have another thing coming in her case. For she realized that if this was indeed cancer, she would be involved in a fight for her life. And in that fight, nobody could tell her what to do. She was on her own. In the short time that had gone by —incredibly it had only been four hours since she had first discovered the tumor—she had done some deep thinking on the matter.

Standing outside the doctors' office, in the gloom of Eighth Avenue, Brooklyn, she and Ralph said good-bye soberly. They had little time—she was going to work, since she knew if she stayed home she would only brood on the problem—and besides, she didn't *feel* sick, quite the contrary: she had not felt better in years!

Ralph sat at the butcher-block kitchen table, a legal-sized pad in front of him. It was seven o'clock. Martha would be starting work. B.J. had called from the city: he was going uptown to try and find some English girl he was dating. Ordinarily, Ralph would have blown up at him: there was a rule—no dating on weekdays. But he had said nothing, relieved that neither kid would be home while he made the telephone calls. They were a close family, in a strange sort of way. There was only twenty years separating them and their children, and they had all been through much together. In a sense they were like contemporaries, no matter how much Martha and Ralph tried to emphasize their authority in the house.

B.J. seemed surprised at Ralph's mild response—"Be home by midnight, you've got school tomorrow."

"Is there anything wrong?" he asked.

"Nothing, really, just some upsetting things happened today. I'll tell you about it when you get home."

"Okay, see you later." B.J. would forget about it by the time he got home. Martha and Ralph didn't want to tell the kids or their parents anything until at least they had spoken to the surgeon.

The next call was to Ellen Greenberg. Ralph and she had gotten close working on a story about the medical consequences of nuclear war. They had become friends, and the two couples had socialized a few times. The Greenbergs were both doctors: Ellen worked in a health-maintenance group, Bill did medical research.

Ellen answered the phone with a perfunctory "Hi."

"Hi, Ellen. This is Ralph."

She was glad to hear from him, she said, but her tone sounded fussy, even a bit annoyed.

"Listen, I've got a problem I thought maybe you could help me with. That is, Martha has a problem."

He knew his voice was shaky, and she could hear it underneath his almost breezy casualness.

"What's the matter?" Ellen almost screamed. She and her husband were alarmists, and it was a private joke between Martha and Ralph to contrast the Greenbergs to the laid-back Kurzes, whom they had known in medical school. Two entirely different styles of medicine. To Ellen, everything was a potential disaster. The lightning bolt was always about to strike. The Kurzes, on the other hand, were of the "take two aspirins" school. Things usually get better by themselves.

"Well, nothing, I hope. It's just that Martha discovered this growth this afternoon. . . ."

"Where? Her breast?" asked Ellen intuitively.

"Yes," said Ralph. He laughed for no particular reason, just nervousness. "She was just showering and, well, there it was. As she said, *it* found *her.*"

Ellen demanded details: what was its size, what did it feel like, where was it located? When he said it was in the upper outside part of the left breast, there was a pause on the other end, a bit of silence. He knew Ellen well enough to know she was disturbed at something.

"What's wrong? What did I say?" he asked.

"Nothing. It's just that for some reason that's the most common site for cancer. We don't know why, but cancer more frequently strikes the *left* breast than the right, and more frequently appears in the upper outer quadrant."

"Strange," said Ralph, struggling to maintain an intellectual detachment from the problem. "I wonder why that is?" He felt a hollowness inside.

"Nobody knows. There's a lot that's not known about breast cancer. And amazingly, very little research has been done on it. I think there's been a kind of male chauvinist aversion to the topic, a failure to take it seriously as a research problem. But that's just my impression."

"Well, the Kurzes don't think it's cancer," said Ralph. He was fishing—he wanted to hear her say it.

"Well, the Kurzes never believe anything is dangerous or important," said Ellen angrily. He could imagine her black eyes flashing. "They're wonderful people, but let's face it, they're Pollyannas. I mean, after all, Martha had checkups recently, right? Why didn't they discover this lump when she went to see them?"

"True, but they—"

"Well, there you are."

"Why are you trying to convince me that Martha has cancer?" His voice came out angry, although the last thing in the world he wanted to do right now was fight with Ellen Greenberg. All he wanted was a reassuring word, but it looked like he had gone to the wrong person.

"I'm not," she said, more moderately. "I just want to make sure you take this seriously. Martha's going to have this looked at by a very competent person. Do you have somebody?"

"We got a referral to a Dr. Leslie Strong," said Ralph.

"I don't know him," said Ellen. It sounded like a condemnation.

"Do you have somebody you'd recommend?" asked Ralph.

"Not for breast, no. Not for breast." Her voice sounded a bit strange.

"So," he said after a pause. "How are things with you? Did Bill get his grant?" Her husband did some kind of cancer research work on cats. He had wanted to work on monkeys, he said, but cats were cheaper.

"No." She dragged the word out, hesitating. "Listen. I'm not supposed to tell you this, but I guess you should know."

There was a portentous air, the leaden feel of disaster.

"Bill's got Hodgkin's disease, Ralph. He doesn't want anybody to know until we get the biopsy results. But it's a classic case, all the symptoms."

"God, Ellen," said Ralph. "I can't believe this." He was really stunned. Bill was five years younger than he. In his mind he tried to call up the statistics on Hodgkin's disease. Was it 80 percent survival after five years, or only 20 percent? In any case, it was terrible. Surgery, radiation, chemotherapy. The whole bit. He suddenly felt very close to Ellen, or wanted to be.

"I've got to run. Baby's crying," said Ellen. "Listen, make sure you look after her. Make sure you get somebody good. Get the best."

"What's going on in the world?" Ralph said. "It seems like everybody's coming down with cancer!"

"Take care," said Ellen, who seemed to regret having opened up to him. "Talk to you in a few days." And she hung up.

Ralph walked around the apartment, turning on lights, shaking his head sadly. The whole world seemed to be coming apart at the seams. Unraveling. He felt that he had to be strong to keep this period of choppy water from sinking the whole boat.

The phone rang.

"Hello. This is Dr. Strong."

Ralph tried to picture the man from the voice. It was a cultured voice, self-assured sounding.

"I understand from Dr. Kurz that your wife has a breast tumor. If you like, I could see her this Wednesday at two P.M."

"First, I'd like to ask you a few questions," said Ralph. He could tell the doctor was busy, but he didn't intend to be rushed.

"Sure," said Strong. "Fire away."

Ralph found a sheet of scrap paper on which he had scrawled some questions.

"First of all, do you do a mastectomy automatically if it's malignant? Or will you be willing to allow it as a separate decision?"

"I *never* do a mastectomy automatically," said Strong. "Only if the patient insists. I do what is called the two-stage procedure.

"The first stage is an excisional biopsy. This is the complete removal of the entire breast tumor. This is then analyzed by frozen section to see if it's malignant," said Strong.

"Would she have to stay overnight for this?" asked Ralph.

"That depends," Strong answered. "If the tumor is superficial, that is, near the surface of the skin, then it can often be done under local anesthesia. If it's deeper, then we have to use general anesthesia, and she should stay in the hospital a few days. She would then go home. Based on the pathology report, I would then discuss the kind of further treatment that might be necessary.

"Most tumors turn out to be benign, especially in women your wife's age. She's forty years old, right? But if it turns out to be malignant, then I'll discuss the *kind* of cancer it is and, based on the kind of problem, we'll try to fashion the correct treatment for this type. Do you understand?"

"I thought that the mastectomy was standard treatment for breast cancer," said Ralph. "What alternatives would we have?"

"Well, the usual treatment for breast cancer today, of all types, is the modified radical mastectomy. But there are two new treatments that have become available recently. The first of these is called a 'quadrantectomy.' The second is a simple 'lumpectomy.' I will discuss these both with you when you come in. But in no case would we do a mastectomy at the same time as the biopsy, unless the patient herself insisted. We want the patient to participate and ask questions, to take part in the decision-making."

"Things have changed a lot since the last time I looked into this question," said Ralph. He had written a story about breast cancer some years back, when Mrs. Rockefeller and Mrs. Ford had had their operations. At that time it was, literally, standard operating procedure to anesthetize the patient only once: if the tumor proved to be cancerous upon biopsy, the surgeons then removed the breast as well. In almost all cases they used the radical Halsted procedure, in which the pectoral muscles were also taken out, to facilitate removal of the lymph nodes. Some doctors went further and recommended a "super-radical" in many cases: this involved removal of the chain of lymph nodes that lay across the breast bone.

"Isn't this limited approach still controversial?" asked Ralph.

"Yes, the quadrantectomy is one of the big controversies in breast treatment," said Strong. "Many of the old guard still refuse to accept it, but little by little the concept of a more sparing, conservative approach is gaining strength. Leaving the muscles for further reconstruction and preventing any kind of deformity have become major goals, at least with us in the Breast Health Program. Any further questions?"

Ralph thought. Of course, there were a million, but they all eventually resolved themselves into one: does his wife have cancer? And only a biopsy would show that. He was generally pleased with Strong's answers so far. They seemed open-minded, if a bit cut and dried. But that's the way surgeons were. It came with the job. He had never met one who was exactly hung loose.

"What hospital would you use if she needed an operation?" Ralph asked.

"Well, she could have her choice. I'm affiliated with Mount Sinai, Beth Israel, and Methodist. Since you live in Brooklyn, I would suggest Methodist."

"How is the pathology department there?" The pathology department would make the final determination whether or not Martha had cancer. The doctor—any doctor—would have to go by their decision, so a slip-up there could be a tragedy.

"They're very good," said Strong. "Any other questions?"

There was an awkward pause. Ralph still hadn't even accepted the fact that Martha would have to go see a surgeon. A surgeon meant cutting, possibly mutilation. Possibly even death. What about their daughter's disastrous operation, which had left her incapacitated by head pains for six months and almost ruined her young life? Yet truly there seemed no way out.

"When did you say she could see you?" Ralph asked finally, and they made a date for Wednesday. It would be a terrible two days.

After they hung up, Ralph sat for a while with his head cradled in his hands on the table. He smiled sadly: sitting like this reminded him of rest period in elementary school, the smell of crayons and other kids' tunafish sandwiches. P.S. 225. 1953. 1954. 1955. It all seemed so very far away now, like another life, like someone else's life.

Martha was sitting in the back room at AutoFont. She sat upright at her machine, a ratty straw hat like something out of *The Wizard of Oz* perched on her head. The fluorescent lights seemed to glare more than usual and she turned up the contrast on the computer screen.

Around her sat six or seven other typesetters—or typographers, the fancier title she used for credit card applications. On her copy stand sat a bulky job ticket. She was scrutinizing the job, a particularly frustrating bit of work. It was an ad for one of the regional telephone companies. It showed a globe. Martha had to shape the text around the globe. This was not a particularly difficult thing for her, or at least not in normal times. But for some reason tonight, it just wasn't working. Each time she put the computer into its hyphenate-and-justify mode, it showed clearly that the line breaks were all wrong. By the third time she was so frustrated she could scream.

"Anyone feel like falafelling?" asked Bernard, the Australian musician whose desk adjoined hers. (For some reason yet unfathomed, musicians seemed to make the best typesetters. Her shop had enough to start a small orchestra.)

"Oh, is anybody going to Falafeland?" asked Janet.

They all laughed, except Martha, who stared grimly into the screen, which was filled with letters, symbols, asterisks, numbers in a mad jumble.

"Bernard's going to get goodies at Tel Aviv Pizza," said Janet, who was her closest friend at work. "Want anything?"

"Listen, stop interrupting me," Martha yelled. "Im trying to get this damn H and J to work—"

She saw the shock on Janet's face and stopped.

"I'm sorry," said Martha, but before she could even apologize, Janet was backing up and saying, "Don't apologize, that's nothing. I shouldn't have bothered you."

Martha glanced around. Everyone was busy with their jobs, but they all were watching her from the corner of their eyes.

She took two deep breaths. "Bernard, if you're going out, would you please get me a bottled water?"

"Sure, no problem," he said sweetly.

The foreman, Paul, came over, prowling around. She had known him for six years, since she had started her typesetting career at a different shop. Martha was the best typesetter on nights, and Paul, who was no slouch himself, sometimes had to come to her for answers. She hated to do it, but now she had to ask his help.

"Paul, I can't seem to get this thing to shape up right."

He leaned over her, his belly brushing against her side. "Beer Drinkers Make Better Lovers," proclaimed his T-shirt.

Paul scrutinized her text, which was, as usual, very clean and ready to send to the background processor, if it weren't for this problem.

"We've been having this problem a lot today, especially on the B system," said Paul. "It won't hyphenate and justify properly. It's a bitch! The thing to do is throw in a lot of 'cancel indents.' Just scatter 'em around. Overkill, I call it. Sometimes the only thing the computer understands is violence. Try that," he said, walking away nonchalantly.

"Damn it, Paul, why the hell didn't you tell me this before I wasted half a goddamned hour on this thing?"

Paul turned slowly. "Huh? What's eating you?" he said, and he walked out of the room.

When Bernard returned from the falafel place she poured herself a glass of cold water. She could call Ralph to find out if the surgeon had phoned and what he had said. She hesitated, because the only telephone was right behind her desk, right out in public. No privacy. She didn't want everyone to know her business, at least not until she went into the hospital, and even then, maybe not. People gossip. Besides, she remembered what happened when another typesetter had gone in to have papillomas removed from his larynx. You could hear the word "cancer" being whispered all over the place, from the service department straight through to the proofreaders' corner. It was like the fear of contagion or something. One typesetter even had insisted on cleaning her work area with Fantastik for half an hour each evening. When asked why, she said, "I *know* that's contagious! That's cancer!" and she kept on scrubbing away at the plastic-topped computer desk.

Suddenly Martha felt ill. She had forgotten to eat dinner and had been running around. Perhaps that was it. The water sat like an ice cube in her stomach.

What to do? It was only her nerves, she thought, just the tension of this terrible day. Take some more water. But more water didn't cure her; it only made her feel worse. Suddenly she noticed something on the side of the bottle: some kind of white deposit.

My God, she thought. I've been poisoned!

She held the bottle up. Sure enough, on the green glass, each time she shook it, little white dots the size of pinheads formed. Was the bottle sealed when she opened it? She couldn't remember. Maybe it wasn't! Maybe someone had slipped some poison into the water, the same way they did with Tylenol in Chicago!

She stood up, but she staggered and held onto the edge of her desk.

"What's the matter?" asked Janet. She had forgotten her anger when she saw how pale Martha was.

"I—I think I'm going to be sick," said Martha. Janet left her machine and helped her to the bathroom.

"I think I've been . . . poisoned," said Martha. "The water."

"Poisoned?" said Janet. "How? I mean, who would want to poison you?"

"Go look at the bottle. Take a look. Maybe I should go to the hospital and they can pump my stomach."

"Let me help you into the lounge and I'll go look at the bottle," said Janet. Martha could tell she didn't believe her, but she appreciated the help. She felt awful, her face cold and sweaty. She was a little better now that she had gotten rid of the water, but felt weak. Martha lay on the grimy plaid couch in the breakroom. Paul came by, poked his head in, and said something. Then he left. One of the messengers looked in on her, too. Finally, Janet came back with the green bottle.

"There's nothing wrong with this bottle," she said. "It says right here on the side that mineral deposits may accumulate at cold temperatures. You should read labels. I'm sure there's nothing wrong with it."

Martha closed her eyelids and her eyes shuddered behind them. "I know," she said slowly. "There's nothing wrong with it. There's something wrong with me, though." She was sobbing now, gently.

Janet sat down on the edge of the couch.

"Something wrong with me, Janet," she blubbered, like a baby. "I have something . . . a growth . . . I'm afraid, Janet. I'm afraid I have cancer!"

Dr. Strong's Brooklyn office was on Prospect Park West, in one of the loveliest sections of the borough. Martha and Ralph were early for their appointment. As they waited, Strong's nurse, Susan Fisherman, gave them copies of the BHP *Bulletin.*

"Dr. Strong will see you now," said Susan.

They found Strong sitting at his desk in his shirtsleeves.

"Hi, come in. Shut the door."

Strong was a man about their own age, which they found somehow reassuring.

"Do you have a family history of breast cancer?" he asked Martha.

"Yes," she said. "My grandmother had breast cancer. That was many years ago." She had thought of this many times since she had discovered the lump just two days before. Was it true that breast cancer ran in families, that it was hereditary? Or was that just another myth—like the one about breast disease being caused by a blow. Or by men fondling your breasts too roughly during sex?

"And your mother?"

"Well, my mother and my sisters all have trouble with their breasts. . . ."

"Trouble?" asked Strong, a bit alarmed.

"Lumps. You know, before their periods. I do too. But nobody has ever had breast cancer. But, Doctor, do you think that this predisposes me to have a malignancy?"

Strong nodded.

"Yes, it's true. Your risk increases. If anyone in your family has a history of breast cancer—on either side, by the way—your risk goes up about three-fold. But if your mother or sister has breast cancer it can go as high as nine times—if the disease occurs before menopause and if it occurs in both breasts at once. Was that the case in your grandmother's disease?"

"I . . . I don't know. But I think it was only in one breast."

"Then there's less of a risk," said Strong. He felt bad for a moment. This woman was obviously scared. What she really wanted was to be reassured, to be told not to worry. Instead, he gave her facts and figures that might possibly alarm her.

"When did you first get your period?" Strong asked.

"When I was twelve," said Martha. "Why is that important?"

"It's another risk factor. The length of time you experience menstruation—what we call 'menarche'—influences your chances of getting breast cancer. Generally speaking, the longer the menarche the greater the chance. Thus, if you began your period at age ten or eleven, and continued to get it into your fifties, you would be at greater risk than a woman who began late and ended early."

"Why is that?" asked Ralph.

"Hormones," said Strong. "The breast is very sensitive to female hormones, and when your wife gets her period she experiences a change in the level of these hormones. This seems to sensitize the breasts to the development of tumors over a long period of time.

"Is there anything else you want to tell me about your breasts?" he asked, after going through all the routine questions. Sometimes he overlooked an important risk factor or clue.

"Well, I've always liked my breasts," she said. Strong laughed. She was very open, warm, and almost childlike, although he sensed she could be tough, as well.

"I was proud of them in junior high school, because I got them before any of the other girls. I thought they were very beautiful," she added.

"They are," said Ralph, and then he quickly felt stupid for having said it.

"On the other hand, I was brought up to be sort of afraid of them. My mother had had to change my grandmother's mastectomy bandages while she herself was a teenager, while her own breasts were coming in. That must have been terrible, and I think she passed on her own fears or phobias or whatever to me. I wasn't able to nurse," she said, and her voice showed Strong that this was a source of anxiety, probably guilt.

"Why was that?" he asked gently.

"Well, I don't know. My mother was present soon after both births and she was always insisting that *I* could never breastfeed, that my nipples were not the right type, that they were 'inverted,' or that I didn't have enough milk."

"Couldn't you just ignore her?" asked Strong.

Ralph laughed.

"My mother is not the kind of person you just ignore, Doctor," said Martha. "I tried, with my daughter, and the hospital was giving her water, but my mother demanded that they give her milk."

"She broke into the nursery and grabbed a bottle out of the nurse's hand," said Ralph quietly. It was one of his favorite memories of his mother-in-law.

"That's very interesting," said Strong, and he meant it. He would have to tell this story to Dr. Gerald Lucas, the psychiatrist who served as consultant to the Breast Health Program. Lucas was interested in all psychological aspects of breast disease. He collected anecdotes of women with breast problems who had unusual psychological experiences with their breasts. While there was no simple one-to-one correspondence, he believed there was such a thing as a "cancer personality," which would predispose toward malignancy.

"When I was twelve," Martha went on, "my father died of a heart attack."

It sounded so immediate in her mind that Strong said, "I'm sorry."

"He was only thirty-three," she said. "He left behind—besides a widow and four daughters—a beautiful Italian accordion. Since I looked like my father, it fell to me to take up the accordion. I learned quickly and each performance would bring a flood of tears and reminiscences. But my breasts were coming in at this time and the accordion irritated them terribly. Finally the doctor ordered me to stop. I guess in the back of my mind I always wondered if I didn't do permanent damage to my breast with that . . . irritation."

"Well, you know that 'irritation' was one of the original theories of cancer. But that's simply not the case. It's a much more complicated disease than that. I think you can rid your mind of the feeling that you may have injured yourself in this way."

"I felt guilty about stopping, though, since it seemed at that age to be a kind of betrayal of my father's memory and of my mother's need to have some living reminder of him. I don't know why I'm telling you all this. It's just that I want you to understand what a tangle of emotions I have connected with my breasts."

"No, I appreciate it," Strong said warmly. "Do you have anything else you want to say? If not, I'd like to examine you."

Ralph had been almost silent till now, scrutinizing Strong and making a study of his diplomas and certificates, as he always did in doctors' offices. It was an impressive collection: American International College, with a Phi Beta Kappa key; an M.D. from the University of California, Los Angeles; first-year residency at Columbia Presbyterian, followed up by four more years of residency at Kings County Medical Center and Downstate Medical Center. After that, Strong had been a clinical instructor in surgery at Brooklyn-Cumberland Medical Center, affiliated with Downstate. He was board-certified, a fellow of the America College of Surgeons, and a member of the New

York Metropolitan Breast Cancer Society, which **Ralph**, as a science writer, knew was the "inner circle" of breast doctors in the New York area. The credentials were obviously all in place, but that didn't answer the ultimate question: was this a person to whom they wanted to entrust Martha's health, and possibly her life?

Ralph unfolded some of his notes gathered over the last two days. Some of them were indecipherable to anyone but himself: on one, for instance, he had written,

>   -Phys
>   -mam
>   -needle
>   -if biop
>   -excisional not
>   -incisional
>   -see as an o.p.

On another he had written:

> incisional biopsy for tumor
> cyst-aspiration
> *don't sign for mastectomy*
> —tremendously traumatic
> —new data—want time to think

That last phrase summed it up. Ralph was an intellectual, with scholarly habits, the type of person who carefully researched the purchase of a toaster oven. But now there was no time to think. He knew that once the cancer (if it was cancer) spread beyond the breast itself, Martha's chances of survival would go way down.

There were so many questions, he thought. But better to wait until Strong made his diagnosis. The doctor and Martha went into the examining room, and Ralph stayed behind to peruse an article by Gerald Lucas in the BHP *Bulletin.*

Inside, Martha removed her blouse and her bra. She felt awkward and vulnerable. She gave a little scream as the doctor approached her and he pulled back, surprised and a bit annoyed.

"I haven't even touched you yet," Strong said, with mock anger. "Calm down! What are you afraid of?"

"I . . . don't like to have my breasts touched."

Strong looked at the ceiling, as if for guidance.

"You're exasperating," he said familiarly. "Just relax, relax. I'm just going to poke around a bit. I'm not going to hurt you." He cupped the left breast gently with one hand, and then pressed in firmly with the other. Martha breathed slowly, deliberately. Once he touched her it wasn't so bad.

The breasts were very lumpy, more lumpy than she probably knew, since she struck him as the ostrich type who rarely if ever examined herself.

In the upper left quadrant he could feel something different than the routine cystic lumps and bumps of her breast. It was larger, smoother, a bit detached from the rest of the breast tissue.

"Is this it? Is this what you found?" he asked softly.

She nodded, her bottom lip caught between her teeth.

His face registered concern. He pressed harder. "You may be a little sore tomorrow morning. Don't be surprised," he said.

She winced.

"Okay, now I would like you to lie down here, on your back." She lay down on the examining table, her face touching the smooth white paper. How she hated that paper, its coolness, its impersonality.

Strong repeated the whole procedure again, this time pressing down on her chest. He then examined the other breast, paying special attention to the mirror-image area.

"Sometimes these problems pop up simultaneously in both breasts, in what we call the contralateral breasts as well." He felt a toughening there, probably a fibrocystic growth, but nothing comparable to the left breast.

"Are you done?" she asked, suddenly feeling a bit claustrophobic and panicky.

"Almost," he fibbed, sensing her anxiety. "I just want to take one more feel. This time from the side." He made her lie on her side and he repeated the whole procedure once more.

"You can feel it, right? Is it, you know, something *bad*?"

"Okay, you can get dressed now," he said, ignoring her question for the moment. "Let's talk in my office, all three of us."

Ralph looked up anxiously when they came in. He was afraid to ask anything. Better let the doctor speak first.

"Well, first of all, you should know that Martha has severe fibrocystic disease," said Strong.

"Disease?" asked Martha, her eyes widening.

"Well, that sounds worse than it really is. What that means is you have very lumpy breasts. From what you say, there's a family history of this. That's common. But this underlying condition makes it hard to maintain good breast health because it makes it quite difficult to detect more dangerous conditions."

"Is that what that big lump is, then?" Martha asked. "Fibrocystic?"

"No, I don't think so," said Strong. "It will be impossible to really tell without an operation. But my judgment is that it is a tumor."

"What kind of tumor?" asked Ralph. He was so worried that with each blink of his eyes the room seemed to move slightly.

"My guess is that it is benign. I say that based on the fact that it moves rather freely and that its boundaries are well delineated. Also, at Martha's age a cancerous tumor would be unusual. I would like her to be admitted to Methodist next Wednesday, however, for a biopsy. Without a biopsy, we can't tell for sure."

Ralph thought of his notes and of his conversation with Ellen Greenberg.

"Couldn't this be handled through an incisional biopsy?"

Strong was a bit surprised at the facility with which Ralph handled medical terms. Unlike many doctors, however, he liked his patients to be well informed.

"No, an excisional biopsy is preferable," said Strong. "It's safer to take out the whole tumor. With an incisional biopsy we remove just a portion, a slice. But that still leaves the problem. You want to remove the whole thing. You can see already that this tumor has pushed the left breast out of shape already. It will keep on growing, almost indefinitely. Besides, cosmetic considerations aside, a tumor like this is dangerous because it can mask other things going on in the breast."

That sounded reasonable to both Martha and Ralph, and they communicated and confirmed this through eye contact, an almost imperceptible sign language worked out over two decades of familiarity.

"And what about aspiration?" asked Ralph.

"Well, if this were a cyst," said Strong, "we could stick a needle in it and draw off the fluid."

Martha winced: the idea was horrible to her, more horrible in some ways, for some reason, than an operation.

"But it's too hard and tough to be simply a cyst, although there may be some cystic fluid involved with it. But if I draw off the fluid and some tough part remains, well, I'd still have to go in and excise it eventually. Do you understand?"

Everything seemed to be inexorably moving toward an operation, surgery one week from that day. Yet somehow it seemed so unreal. Did she really *need* this operation? Everyone had heard about unnecessary surgery, surgery done more for the sake of the doctor than the patient. Ralph had once heard it defined as a "cashectomy," or the "surgical removal of the wallet." Strong seemed nice, and honest, but who was to say? Maybe this was all a ruse to get her to the operating table.

It reminded him a bit of shopping for a computer. Whom did you listen to, whom did you trust? They had put off a home computer decision for over a year now, and it was no great loss. But this was a decision that couldn't wait. Martha's life might hang in the balance.

"One more question," said Ralph. "What about the effect of the biopsy? I mean, how disfiguring will it be?"

Strong, surprisingly, laughed.

"What's so funny?" asked Ralph, beginning to get angry.

"Your choice of words," said Strong. Ralph calmed down when he saw that Strong was really amused, not just being patronizing. "Disfiguring. Next you'll ask me how 'mutilating' it will be. We have ways of sewing her up again so that you'll hardly know we were there. Special sutures that dissolve slowly, but form scar tissue around them, so that it fills up the hole. I'll explain it all to you both after the surgery."

"What about a scar?"

"It should be minimal."

There was an awkward pause. Strong had made his offer, he didn't want to push. Ralph was afraid to make such a momentous decision for his wife, as much as he was tempted to. Finally Martha said, "Okay, let's get it over with." Ralph could tell she really meant it and that she felt good about Strong. And at least it would be over with. Another bad week, but then, come what may, at least they would *know*. Whatever it was, they could face it together.

They had passed Methodist Hospital a hundred times and never noticed it. When their son was younger he had attended the Montessori Academy down the block. But they barely gave the sprawling hospital complex a second glance. It was less visible than the old armory on Eighth Avenue. If anything, they might have wondered in a vague way what a Methodist hospital was doing in such a heavily Catholic neighborhood as lower Park Slope. It didn't seem like a place they would ever visit. Now, suddenly, their lives were tied up with this institution. Its various buildings, old and new, became important to them. As they waited to be called to the admitting office, they scrutinized the many plaques on the wall, studied the selection of paperbacks in the gift shop, chatted with the ladies in pink.

Mostly they sat on the molded plastic seat and waited, trying to avoid the cigarette smoke of the other people waiting. It was a cross-section of Brooklyn, mostly large families on vigils. A lot of these people seemed inured, as if they had spent much of their lives in hospitals and hospital waiting rooms. They spoke of doctors and nurses. Martha carried her suitcase, which looked a bit pathetic, and hugged her own down pillow she had brought from home. She couldn't sleep without it, like a favorite teddy bear, Ralph thought. He admired her independence, however, in bringing it—it was a smart thing to do. Something familiar, soft, and warm.

She went through the admitting interview without incident. They took an impression of her medical insurance card and fastened a plastic bracelet around her arm. She seemed somehow proud of it. They brought a wheelchair and even though she was not really *sick*, or at least did not feel sick, the orderly made her sit in it for the ride up in the elevator. From that moment she felt a subtle change in her relationship to the hospital. She was in their hands for the duration of her stay. In a funny way, it would be a pleasant feeling to surrender her independence this way, to be totally in the care (and at the mercy) of these strangers, who seemed to know what to do with her better than she knew herself.

But deep down she was in charge and she knew it. She was

undergoing this operation because *she* wanted to. No one could have made her if she hadn't. And she had it all worked out in her mind. If it was cancer, she knew what she was going to do. She would fight for her life. There were basically two paths open to her. She could keep on working and live by her doctor appointments. But she had heard about too many people who had been good little girls and boys and who had also died on schedule. Or she could take charge. She knew that would entail plenty of fighting—with Strong, with her mother and her in-laws, even with Ralph. But she wasn't afraid to fight. In fact, she liked it. She would quit her job and begin a worldwide search for a cure for cancer. She had no doubt, either, that she would find it. She had heard about unorthodox clinics in Mexico, Jamaica, Germany. She would visit them all, even though she knew it would bankrupt her and Ralph to do so. But she would not go down without a terrific fight.

The head nurse, Marie, dropped by in the evening.
"How you getting on?" she asked. "Everything okay?"
"I'm all right," said Martha. "The noise finally stopped."
The nurse laughed. "That can't be helped, I'm afraid. We try to keep it to a minimum."
"What's going on?"
"They're putting up the new wing of the hospital. We're really proud of it. Methodist's a community hospital; it serves a particular geographic area—mainly the Park Slope and Brooklyn Heights areas. It's always been a good place—it's a teaching affiliate of Downstate Medical Center, for instance. But it's gotten a little, well, run down, over the years. Then some influential people got interested in making it a top-flight place again."
"I'm sure it'll be beautiful," said Martha. "But I hope I never have occasion to find out firsthand."
In the morning, early, they woke her. A nurse shaved under her arms. As part of her private plan, for fifteen minutes before the sedative, she touched her toes and did jumping jacks by the side of her bed. If she had thought to bring her jumprope, she would have done that. The nurses looked at her skeptically, but she ignored them. There was a reason for this regimen: a close friend of the family had died a few months before of complications following surgery. She had gone in for a minor operation

and had developed a blood clot in the lungs and simply died. She was only forty-four, just a few years older than Martha herself. Martha believed that exercise would improve her circulation. She intended to do the same thing as soon as she could *after* the operation. If Strong objected, that would be too bad on him. She also took a large dose of vitamins, including A, C, and E. She believed this would help with the healing process as well as the general stress of surgery.

At 8:30 she was lying, sedated, in the corridor of the operating room. Everything seemed dull, but pleasantly so. She realized the drug was beginning to take effect. A man in a mask came by.

"Everything's going to be fine," he said. It was Dr. Strong. She smiled and he pressed her hand.

By nine o'clock he was ready to begin surgery.

The anesthesiologist was warm and friendly.

"I want you to count from twenty for me," he said. "Count backward."

She started to do so, while he added something to the I.V. drip in her arm. She reached thirteen and then stopped. She didn't know why she stopped. The reason was that she was unconscious. She remembered thinking, "Thirteen, unlucky." She tried to go backward at least one more number, one click of the roulette wheel, but the wheel wouldn't turn. She struggled desperately for twelve. But nothing happened. A bad omen, she thought, and fell into a deep, comalike sleep.

After the operation, two orderlies came by and wheeled her down the corridor to the recovery room.

It was a large area with bright sunlight filtering through the windows. Patients were along the walls in movable beds. Doctors and nurses scurried back and forth.

Leslie Strong stood by her bed. Her eyelids fluttered and he reached out and felt her pulse, more as a gesture of friendship and solidarity than out of medical necessity.

Martha opened her eyes. She was barely conscious. "What was it?" she asked, her lips dried, caked, and parched.

"Benign," Strong said, emphasizing each syllable. The nicest word in the English language, he thought.

Martha burst into tears. She sobbed so loudly that three or four nurses and nurses' aides, drinking coffee out of Parthenon-decorated cups, looked up.

Strong felt good. "Now rest, dear. I'll come by and see you later."

The coffee looked good to him. He pulled off his green mask and booties and made his way to the doctors' lounge, sinking into a big leather chair. He had an hour or so before he had to get to the Brooklyn office to see a full schedule of patients there. He closed his eyes and listened to the chatter of the other doctors, mostly shop talk. He was glad about Martha. Very glad. He would have hated to have to tell her otherwise. Sometimes, occasionally, life turned out the way you wanted. Too bad it couldn't always be that way. His anger welled up momentarily as he thought of the many women Martha's age who had not been so fortunate. But what could he do? He had discussed this many times with Dr. Lucas, his analyst friend. All he could do was treat these women the best he could, try to get them to come in for treatment while there was still time. That was why he had founded the Breast Health Program, why he did not hesitate to talk to reporters or to go on television and radio with his message: don't be afraid of your breasts. Take care of their *health* the same way you protect the health of every other part of your body. He thought again of the grim statistics: one out of twelve women would contract breast cancer sometime in her lifetime—114,000 a year in the United States alone. The figures were staggering. A recurrent image popped into his head. When he was in medical school, at the University of California, Los Angeles, he went to a couple of football games. He also got caught in a couple of massive post-game traffic jams as well. Yet U.C.L.A.'s Coliseum, the largest stadium in the country, only held 105,000 people. That meant you could fill the Coliseum with breast cancer victims and still leave 9,000 people sitting in the aisles—and that was one year's group alone! Yet each one of these suffered through her own personal tragedy, her own hell of torment, doubt, and too often crushing defeat. Sometimes, too, he felt as if nobody really cared, that this terrible disease, which still killed two-thirds of its victims, was accepted as a matter of course. The tendency was there in all of us, of course, to *adapt*, no matter how bad the situation. But it was a tendency we had to fight or else no progress could be made in medicine or in life.

It was because of these grim statistics that Strong was a firm believer in mammography. Mammography, or the use of diagnostic X rays of the breast, was the mainstay of the early detection of breast disease.

His mind lingered on the Breast Health Program. It was still young and relatively small. The real test would be if women like Martha came into it. A few people like that could do much to spread the idea of preventive care for the breast. He would make a point of asking her when he went to see her.

Sunk in thought, Strong didn't realize that Ralph had come in and was standing next to him.

"They told me that it was okay to talk to you here," said Ralph. He felt awkward: he had been to many hospitals, but had never been inside a doctors' lounge before. The inner sanctum of the hospital. He imagined the other doctors giving him hostile glances—a layman in our lair—and was even prepared for Strong to blow up at him and order him out at once! Actually, Strong had given instructions for Ralph to be sent to meet him here.

"Sit down," he said, motioning to a leather couch, grown smooth and almost springless from so many weary doctors' rumps.

"Well, good news," said Strong, and Ralph let his breath out. He felt as if he had been holding it for weeks. "It's benign. And it was huge! Incredible. Almost seven inches from end to end."

"How can that be?" asked Ralph.

"Well, it was attached at one end to the chest wall."

"What exactly was it?"

"Well, we'll have to wait for the final pathology report in a couple of days. According to the frozen section, however, it was something unusual. A benign fibroadenoma embedded within a fibrocystic growth. You see, that's why it is so important for her to control that fibrocystic disease of hers. Because tumors can easily hide within them and then you miss them upon examination."

"What causes this?" asked Ralph. It was bewildering.

"Nobody really knows. More research has to be done on it,"

he said, although he knew deep down that not enough research *was* being done.

A nurses' aide wheeled the bed back to room 224. Martha opened her eyes. She was going to ask, "Where am I?" when she suddenly remembered: the hospital. I've had an operation. She could feel the bandage on her chest and make out a tube running out of it. Beyond that she knew nothing. The earlier conversation with Dr. Strong was as if it had never happened.

"What did they find? Did they . . .?"

"I don't know," said the nurses' aide. "All I know is—" she thought back to the scene in the recovery room, the sight of the doctor bending over the bed "—he told you something in recovery. And you burst into tears." Martha moved her parched lips. But no sound came out. She couldn't remember any such conversation, but, then, the whole world was still a fog.

"My God," she whispered and she suddenly felt—no, she *knew*—that the news had been bad. She tried to feel for her breast.

"You rest now," said the aide. "Doctor'll be by later to talk to you, I'm sure."

"Did they remove my breast?" asked Martha desperately.

Just then Ralph got off the elevator and joyfully ran toward the room. He had been waiting for her for almost two hours and had just gone down to make a phone call when she had been wheeled up.

He was a bit frightened when he saw her; she looked so deathly pale, so drained of her vitality. If her hair had suddenly turned white, he would hardly have been more surprised than by this transformation.

"What happened?" she whispered. "What went wrong? The nurse told me—"

"Everything's okay," said Ralph, elated, holding her clammy hand. "I just spoke to Strong. It's benign. Entirely benign."

Martha started to cry, sobbing silently.

"But the nurse just told me I was crying," she said, her brown eyes flooded with soft tears.

"You were crying for *joy*, when the doctor told you the good news," said Ralph. "Just like you are now. It was huge. But he said the incision was small and wouldn't leave a big scar at all."

"Thank God it's over," said Martha. "Are you sure? Are you positive?"

"I'm sure," he said, laughing. "Totally benign."

"Then I'm going to sleep," she said, and in that instant she fell asleep with a smile on her face and her head on her own down pillow.

Mildred

Leslie Strong was running late that Wednesday morning. He slipped into his greens, pausing briefly to admire the panorama of downtown Brooklyn from the bank of windows in the mens' dressing room. The trees were beginning to burst into foliage and the sunlight glinted off the waters of New York's vast harbor.

"Incredible day," he said cheerfully to a cluster of men, all of them surgeons, who were standing around in their underwear beside the lockers. Taping his watch and wallet into his top pocket, he passed through the nurses' lounge and hurried down to the eighth floor, pausing at the door to put on a pair of paper booties from a box by the entrance.

Downstairs he checked the day's schedule. He was doing Nancy Browne first, at nine o'clock. Then Mildred Rosenbloom. Eileen Harrow was supposed to scrub with him. He winced and wondered briefly if someone down in administration was out to get him.

In operating room #5 they were doing vascular surgery, an aortal-femoral bypass. They had been at it since seven-thirty, a cluster of physicians around their bespectacled chief.

"Your first patient is in the hall, Dr. Strong," said the nurse behind the desk. The patients awaiting surgery were on rolling beds outside the operating rooms. He found his, Nancy Browne, and touched her arm. She was drowsy from the premed, but gave him a beautiful smile.

"Don't worry," he said. "Everything will turn out fine. You'll see."

"Promise me you won't do a mastectomy," she said, a bit urgently.

He explained over and over again that it was *he* who insisted on a two-stage procedure for all his patients—first a biopsy and then, if it was malignant, further treatment. There were at least ten different kinds of breast cancer, and each one called for different treatments. In the past ten years, the management of breast disease had really opened up. Yet still they seemed skeptical. He wondered briefly if he was doing something wrong, if somehow he could manage to gain these doubters' confidence. The answer, he knew, lay elsewhere. Ten years before, breast surgeons routinely did a one-stage procedure, and a woman going in for breast surgery didn't know if she would wake up with two, one, or even no breasts. Women's liberation and good medical sense had changed all that, but the public still tended to think of breast surgeons as ruthless and unfeeling.

"Everything will be all right," he repeated. "Are you taking any medication for your thyroid?" There was no indication in the chart.

"Nothing at all," she said sleepily.

Thyroid enlargement had been her original complaint. She had gone to a doctor with whom Strong shared his Brooklyn office, and he had discovered the breast lump and sent her next door.

"I'm not worried, Dr. Strong," Nancy said, and she slowly closed her eyes.

Nancy's problem, he was quite sure, was a fibroadenoma. She was twenty-six years old and these benign growths in the breast were not uncommon in women that age. She also had cysts. These were routinely treated through aspiration. He had done this twice but each month she was back with more fluid.

No one knew what caused these benign problems, although there were theories. Diet seemed to have something to do with it. The consumption of coffee, tea, and chocolate may aggravate the condition. Hormones. Heredity. Meanwhile, the best thing to do was to make a small opening and remove the source of the problem. If all went well, the problem might clear up after that. Sometimes (and this was the part he usually didn't tell the patient) it didn't, and the woman faced a long series of breast biopsies that might leave her breast looking like tic-tac-toe.

The first crisis: Eileen Harrow, the second-year resident who was supposed to scrub with him, had disappeared. He glanced at the clock: surgery was scheduled to begin seven minutes before. Nancy had been wheeled into the operating room and moved onto the table, her arms outstretched. The anesthesiologist was grumbling in his baritone: "Let's get going here. Let's get going." He had a lot of cases, but he was making everybody nervous.

Strong tore open a scrub pack and washed his arms and hands vigorously with disinfectant over the sink. He poked his head into the O.R. but Harrow still hadn't shown. He was starting to get worried. A surgeon *must* have an assistant, a backup person to hold the retractors and do the other routine but necessary chores. This service was usually provided by the residents, would-be surgeons who had completed their M.D.s and internships, but now wanted to be surgeons themselves. They had to complete a three-year program of postdoctoral study before they could go out on their own. (In practice, most of them went on for further study in some subspeciality.)

Eileen Harrow, quite simply, hadn't made it. She had just been informed by the head of the department that her contract wasn't being renewed. After two years she would be going home to Arizona with eternal bitterness toward this hospital and quite possibly, Strong thought, the profession.

At 9:10 A.M., the anesthesiologist's grumbling was turning into a low growl. Harrow had still not shown.

"Will you scrub with me, Yvonne?" Strong asked.

The younger of the two O.R. nurses contemplated the question. She liked Dr. Strong, as much as it could be said that she liked *any* surgeon. But she was wary.

"Okay," she said finally, "but I'm not a technician."

"What's that supposed to mean?" asked Strong.

"I'm not a tech," she repeated heatedly. "I can't work by the book."

Somehow he had stepped on her toes, offended her professional pride. This wasn't hard to do, since some O.R. nurses were as skill-proud and arrogant as the surgeons they worked for.

"I didn't say you were a technician," Strong articulated carefully. "I just asked if you would scrub with me. Harrow hasn't—"

Just then Eileen Harrow came waltzing in. She was a strong-looking woman, with an unusual combination of blond hair and deep brown eyes. Her chin was prominent and thrust forward in a defiant gesture.

"I was in the bathroom."

It was like a junior high school excuse, Strong thought.

"The bathroom!" said Estelle, the older O.R. nurse. "Don't you know you've got surgery fifteen minutes ago? You've been keeping the doctors waiting."

"I figured it wouldn't start on time."

"*Oy vey,*" said Strong, and everybody laughed. But underneath he was trying to figure out how to deal with this. He would have liked to tell her off, but he felt sorry for her, and besides, he could hardly afford to have her walk out. The anesthesiologist was sounding like an angry bull. Nancy was half-anesthetized already. "Please scrub quickly," he said finally. "And let's get going. We have another case besides."

Strong uncovered the patient. Her bronze body was slim, girlish, and as beautiful as her face. They quickly covered her over with disposable blue sheets. Her breasts were vigorously scrubbed and then daubed with a Betadine solution till they glistened yellow on her brown body.

Strong positioned the two overhead lights and with Harrow finally (thank God!) stationed opposite him and the two O.R. nurses to his right he was ready to begin. Even the anesthesiologist stopped making noises and a theatrical hush fell over the room.

"We'll start with the scalpel," Strong said.

He made a self-assured incision, about three inches long and just deep enough to slice through the layers of skin and expose the flesh underneath. A line of thick red blood oozed from the wound about one second later and the resident daubed it up with a gauze pad, then flipped it into a plastic-lined bucket. He then cut deeper.

"Bovie," he said, and the nurse handed him a small instrument with an orange plastic handle.

He held a scalpel in one hand and tried to convey the current to the wound by touching the electric knife to the metal.

"Juice," he said.

The nurse turned up the electrical current on the machine, but nothing happened.

"Juice!" he yelled.

"It's not working, Doctor," the older nurse said quietly.

"I don't believe this!"

"We just had it fixed," said the younger nurse. "We've got another one in the corner," and she rushed over and wheeled it into position.

"Well, back to the 1950s," said Strong, referring to the benighted times when these wonderful instruments were not in general use. "Eileen, tie off by hand where I tell you to." They began the tedious process of tying off the bleeders—small severed arteries—with fine surgical thread.

"Okay, try it again, Doctor," said the older nurse.

The current suddenly sizzled and cauterized a small piece of the wound. A puff of bluish smoke rose between the two doctors.

Cut, dig, burn. Cut, dig, burn. Centimeter by centimeter he went deeper into the hole, careful to keep it as small and as neat as possible. That would be important later on when Nancy looked in the mirror. A small biopsy on the outside of the breast, like this one, would be virtually invisible in six months.

Cut, dig, burn some more. The only sound was the electronic equipment that monitored her vital signs. The anesthesiologist had gone on to another case down the hall but had left his resident in charge, a quiet Chinese with a rather incongruous twenty-four-carat "Credit Suisse" bar around his neck. He squeezed the black bag that kept her breathing. The whirr of the generator was followed by a hiss, as the electric knife cut away another piece of flesh, sealed off another bleeder. (Strong could do either with the flick of his thumb.) A little deeper now.

"There it is," he said excitedly. The tumor came into view. To an untrained eye, however, it was difficult to distinguish from the surrounding white-and-yellow tissue (mostly ducts and fat) of the breast. To Strong, after years of such surgery, it stood out clearly.

"I see it," said Harrow slowly.

"Okay, grab hold of it, but gently. See if you can coax it out."

"Damn!" said Harrow sharply through the mask. Her brown eyes flashed.

The two O.R. nurses looked at each other—they were used to communicating with their eyes only. They had made up their minds about Eileen Harrow a long time ago. The story about her lateness would be all over the floor by lunchtime.

"I can't seem to get a hold of it," said Harrow.

"That's okay," said Strong. "Just take it slow . . . and easy." He took the instrument from her and showed her how. "It's very friable, you see. It just falls apart to the touch. That's a characteristic of many of these fibroadenomas." He took the clamp in one hand, the scalpel in the other, and gently coaxed the bulk of the tumor free.

"Cut here . . . and here," he instructed, and she cut. "We're a good team together, Eileen," he said. "You're good." It wasn't all ego reinforcement, either. He basically liked Eileen Harrow, admired her real concern for the patients and the skill that was beginning to flow from it. But at medical politics she got an F.

She didn't acknowledge the compliment—ever her gracious self. Make that an F-minus.

"Cut a good margin around it," he said. "Always take a margin." This was something you learned from day one. That way, if by some chance it turns out to be cancer, you haven't left any stray bits and pieces around to start further tumors.

As each piece of the growth came out he gently deposited it in a metal tray. This was then covered over. In the hallway a messenger from the pathology department was hanging out with some fellow Jamaicans. Their laughter could be heard in the operating room, lightening the atmosphere.

"Do you want a frozen section on this, Dr. Strong?" he asked.

Strong always wanted frozen sections, a technique for examining tissue that results in rapid diagnoses. The tissue is first frozen in liquid nitrogen and then shaved by a machine called a microtome. The reports are usually ready in about fifteen minutes. Paraffin (wax) sections, while more definitive and a bit more reliable, took a couple of days of laborious procedures.

"Frozen, plus estrogen and progesterone receptors."

"Is the estrogen receptor a sign of cancer?" asked Yvonne, the younger O.R. nurse.

Strong was a bit surprised by the question—he thought nurses learned this stuff in school—but he was happy to teach her as well.

"Estrogen and progesterone are female hormones. Sometimes hormones can affect the growth of tumors. We have tests to see if the tumor tissue is affected by these hormones. These tests are called the ERA, or estrogen receptor assay, and the PGRA, or progesterone receptor assay. If the tumor is sensitive to the hormones, then prognosis for the patient is somewhat better. Hormone-dependent tumors are more easily killed by chemotherapy. Also, it opens up alternative avenues of treatment. For instance, we can then use a drug called tomoxifin, which is an anti-estrogen. So, in general, the patient is better off with a positive response, if she has cancer."

"The big if," said the nurse.

"There's the chest wall," said Strong. He reached a gloved finger into a neatly hollowed hole. He cleaned out the hole with a piece of gauze, which the nurse then took from him. Harrow leaned over and peered straight through the hole clear down to the grayish muscle of the chest. Strong took a large plastic syringe and irrigated the hole with disinfectant.

"I think she's going to be okay," said Strong. It was 9:50. The whole procedure had taken less than half an hour.

"Let's sew her up. I'll let you do this one, Eileen. As far as I know she's not a keloid-former and so she should have a nice, neat scar." (Some of his black patients formed keloid scars, which made surgery traumatic and reconstruction, when necessary, more difficult.)

"I know how," said Eileen. "You showed me last time." She swallowed and took her first stitch, deep inside the hole. She worked back and forth from one side to the other. Eventually some normal scar tissue would form around these stitches. The stitches would dissolve, but the scars would remain. The body would have closed in around the hole. Otherwise, there could be an unsightly dip in the woman's breast.

When Eileen's hand reached the surface of the wound, Strong guided her.

"You do it this way—don't leave any crosshatching at all on the skin itself." She took a stitch with the curved needle into the red rim just below the skin.

"Good," said Strong. "But watch that you don't touch the skin over there. Now crossways, over there. Watch out. Good. Very good."

"I know that. And you know that. But no one else seems to."

They were done. Strong stepped away and pulled down the top of his face mask. "I know it's hard to be a woman in surgery, Eileen, but you've got to learn to play the game. At least till you get past your residency."

"I speak my mind. If something's wrong I say so."

"Like turning in the chief resident," said Yvonne, laughing.

The anesthesiologist disconnected his equipment. Nancy was stirring slightly. She looked peaceful.

"That's right," said Eileen. "He was in the wrong."

Strong shook his head. "Well, I admire your chutzpah. Good luck, Eileen."

How Not to Succeed at Surgery, he thought. Few professions were as structured, as hierarchical and conservative as this one. Women in surgery was a revolution. And yet what a pity and a waste that Eileen couldn't find her way through that minefield.

"Please write it up," said Strong, handing her the chart. "And be back here by 10:20, promptly. We've got another case on tap. A serious one."

He let out his breath in the hall. Nancy Browne, pushed by two orderlies, disappeared around the corner into post-op. It had gone as planned. A successful operation was always a pleasure, a relief. The hard one was coming up next.

Strong strolled down the corridor. He could see that every surgical room was occupied. In #2, an older surgeon, who had been his own professor at Downstate, was about to operate on a beautiful tiny baby, maybe six weeks old. It looked so out of place in that big operating room under the glare of the lamps.

Around the corner Strong ran into the pathologist.

"Just the man I'm looking for," said Strong. "Did you get the results on that last patient? Nancy Browne?"

"I took a quick peek," said the other doctor. "Looks like a

fibroadenoma. I'll know for sure in a few minutes. Got more cases today?"

"One more, Mildred Rosenbloom. A mass in the right breast, palpable axillary nodes, skin retraction."

The pathologist, a kindly man, winced. They both knew it was almost certainly cancer.

"Well, maybe it'll turn out okay. I'm starving. Gonna go grab something to eat."

Ten minutes till he began on Mildred. Strong made his way into the anesthesiologist's lounge. Four or five men sat silently in the small room. An air of what might be described as "battle fatigue" hung over the assembly. Strong poured himself a cup of coffee and helped himself to a few cookies, the best in the hospital.

His ten minutes went by quickly. When he returned to the O.R. they were wheeling Mildred in. Harrow was there—her interest in the case battling her determination to get even somehow with the hospital.

"Hello, Mildred," he said, from behind his green mask. "Don't worry, dear. Everything's under control."

He and Eileen went to the view box on the far end of the operating room to study the mammograms of Mildred that had just been taken. Strong put the X rays up on the board. "You see this area here," he said, touching a milky-white area just behind the nipple?

"CA?"

"You can't really tell just by mammography," said Strong. "But it all adds up to mammary carcinoma, doesn't it? It's classic. She's had skin retraction and dimpling for months now. We're going to do an incisional biopsy, and take some of the axillary nodes as well. She's a wonderful woman, but it would have to be a miracle for this not to be cancer."

They "prepped" Mildred as they had her roommate, Nancy, before her. When they uncovered her briefly, Strong was surprised to see how youthful her body was. It moved him with a deep feeling of sympathy and pity.

He held out his hands and Yvonne put the thin, almost transparent gloves on them, overlapping the cuffs of his green coat. "Left hand first," the nurse yelled—her idiosyncrasy an operating room joke.

Then, when the anesthesiologist gave the nod, he made a circular incision underneath the nipple and proceeded to remove the tumor.

The conversation, meanwhile, was surprisingly, almost incongruously light.

"You know," Yvonne said, "that woman you did yesterday is somehow related to that gal down in intensive care. . . ."

"Which one?" said the older nurse, suddenly interested.

"The one with the Mariel Hemingway look."

They were interrupted by the static from the intercom system. The O.R.s were connected with the pathology department, on the second floor, by these devices, which were equipped with speakers. The problem was that there was a lot of background noise in the O.R. and the voices were invariably fuzzy.

"That patient of yours, Strong, that was invasive medullary carcinoma. . . ."

Strong put down his instruments and went to the speaker.

"Say that again, please."

"Browne . . . that was medullary CA, Strong."

There was a look approaching horror in Leslie Strong's eyes—like watching someone being run down by a truck.

"You *must* be mistaken," he yelled. "You mean Rosenbloom—the latest sample I sent down?" But in his guts he knew that the pathologist wasn't mistaken. He rarely was.

"No mistake, Strong. I haven't even analyzed Rosenbloom yet. I'm talking about your first patient, Nancy Browne. B-R-O-W-N-E." Some more static. ". . . the youngest we've ever seen of this type in the hospital. Twenty-six years old."

The speaker went dead, and Strong returned slowly to Mildred, who slept silently on the table.

He thought about Nancy. This kind of cancer, medullary carcinoma, comprised between 5 and 7 percent of breast carcinomas. As the textbooks said, they tended to appear in the young. How terrible it is, however, when "the young" is a beautiful young woman you happen to know and like.

All the normal chatter had ceased.

"And she was such a lovely person, too," said Eileen, unconscious of using the past tense.

"I just can't believe this!" Strong said with determination. "I can't believe it! How the hell am I going to tell her this? Her family. Her boyfriend. Twenty-six years old. Do you realize what this means? Maybe there was a mistake. No, there was no mistake," he answered himself. "And it's in the upper outer quadrant," he said to Eileen—imploringly, not professorially. "The nodes are probably involved."

"Involved nodes" meant the cancer had spread out of its original site—it is no longer simply a 'local' disease but has become "regional." If it had also spread beyond the region, which is basically the armpit into which the breast's lymphatic vessels drain, then it became "systemic." It had then spread throughout the whole body.

This distinction between "local," "regional," and "systemic" was the key to the treatment of breast cancer. If the disease was exclusively local, then it could usually be treated with the removal of a quarter of the breast in which the tumor occurred—a quadrantectomy. This was then followed up by radiotherapy to the breast as a whole. The woman could then be reconstructed, usually with excellent results. On the other hand, if the cancer had already spread to the region, then a modified radical mastectomy was necessary. Also, more extensive radiation and chemotherapy were called into action. It was the oncologist, with his chemotherapeutic agents, who mainly dealt with the systemic aspects of the disease. Nancy would really be in for it.

Something else suddenly occurred to him: her thyroid was enlarged! The cancer could already have spread there. Or there could be another primary tumor in the thyroid, sometimes seen in such cases.

"It's hard to grasp," he said, as he mechanically sewed up Mildred. "Yesterday I had a patient eighty-two years old and she's fine. But poor Nancy . . . It's unfair. Unfair!" he yelled to no one in particular.

"Life is unfair," Yvonne said quickly.

"I know," he said angrily. "But this is *still* unfair."

Mildred awoke to the sound of sobbing. For a moment she thought she had been crying in her sleep, but the sound came from the neighboring bed.

"What's the matter?" she asked drowsily.

Nancy Browne didn't answer.

"What's wrong?" asked Mildred, lifting herself painfully on one elbow. "Should I call the nurse?"

Nancy shook her head. Suddenly it dawned on Mildred.

"They told you you have cancer?" Mildred asked. Nancy nodded.

"I'm okay now. It was just . . . such a surprise. I mean, I'm twenty-six years old."

"Maybe they made a mistake?" asked Mildred, but she knew that that was highly unlikely. Decisions like this were checked and double-checked.

"They said I was the youngest ever in this hospital with this type of disease," said Nancy. With a trace of bitterness she added, "Great, I'll make the record books."

"I had bad news, too," said Mildred. "Mine's also cancer. But I'm trying to live with it. I intend to go on with my life. You can do the same thing."

"But it's not the same thing," said Nancy. "You're old and I'm young." (Mildred wasn't exactly "old," but didn't want to start an argument.) "You've got a husband. Family. You can't compare the two situations."

"God," Mildred sighed. "It's very unfair. But don't worry. Dr. Strong will take good care of you. Did he tell you what kind of operation you would need?"

"Well, he tells me I might be able to have that quadrant operation if my glands are not involved. It's the latest thing. Says it would leave me looking fairly normal. But I've decided I'm going my own way."

"Which is?" asked Mildred.

"I'm going to the top. It's not normal for a twenty-six-year-old woman to get cancer. And if it's spread to the lymph glands besides, I've got to get the *best* doctors on my team."

"Dr. Strong is the best," Mildred said loyally.

"But where do the presidents and vice-presidents send their wives? That's exactly where I'm going to go. This is something very difficult. Don't you understand? I'm fighting for my life here. And not only am I going to the biggest cancer center, but I'm going to get the chairman of the department. I don't want some resident operating on me."

"What do you think they're going to do for you that Dr. Strong can't do? He has access to the same up-to-date information that your cancer center has. There aren't any secrets in this business."

Nancy sighed and hugged her arms to herself. Mildred could tell that she was frightened and, in a controlled way, almost hysterical. She had heard that at the big cancer centers they often went in for very radical surgery. This poor girl might have a more extensive operation than she bargained for once she put herself in their hands. Yet in a way she couldn't help admiring Nancy's gumption. It wasn't easy to wrench yourself away from your doctor and walk into another hospital, a stranger, a complete unknown. Nancy had seemed so meek and unassuming when she had first met her. But obviously this young woman had reservoirs of strength Mildred had hardly suspected.

"I wish you well," said Mildred finally. Something disapproving must have come out in her tone, however, for Nancy said: "I'm not trying to insult Dr. Strong or to insult your choice. But I've got to follow my own path. I don't know that much about medicine. But I know I'm fighting for my life now and the cards are stacked against me. If death is coming, then come on with it. But at least I can meet it fighting, standing on my own two feet!"

PART THREE
Summer

Robin

Robin's vacation came none too soon. She and Peter spent two glorious weeks on Fire Island, where they had shares in a ramshackle summer house. Now it was time to return to the grind, and the future seemed a bit uncertain. The recession was taking its toll: Court Street, where she had tended bar and emceed for almost four years, was about to close. The tips there had been good and the hours suited her perfectly: 8:00 P.M. to 4:00 A.M., Fridays and Saturdays. In those sixteen hours she made more than most secretaries make in thirty-five or forty. In fact, Robin had never worked "normal" hours and pitied people who did. She had always walked to work. Now she might have to take a job with longer hours and lower pay. The prospect was depressing. Nor were singing or dancing gigs easy to find. She had had one, in the *Bugs Bunny Follies.* It wasn't something you bragged about on your résumé.

But she was feeling glorious—tanned, her brown hair now blond-streaked by the sun. She and Peter were getting along fine, not bickering the way they did in the neurotic city. Wouldn't it be great if I hit it big? she thought. Then they could have a house out here all to themselves, or even in the Hamptons, and come out here whenever they wanted. . . .

"Hey, babe, how about a swim? Get into your suit."

The sun was already almost setting and she had to start preparing dinner, but she thought, what the hell, and so ten minutes later (the lobsters having been tucked into their sugar bags in the communal fridge) she and Pete were jogging around in the briny deep. She felt like a kid again, so relaxed, the way she had felt when she went to the Cape with her parents years back. She floated out beyond the breakers and let her mind drift with her body. After half an hour of this therapy she fought her way inshore and found Peter already lying on the blanket. The nearest other couple was a good half mile down the clean white beach. Peter put his arms around her and started to massage her gooseflesh.

"Better get out of your wet clothes," he said.

"In open daylight? Are you crazy?" but she was flattered by his attention. He usually wasn't that demonstrative.

"Crazy for you," he said, and he nuzzled his unshaven face into her neck. Suddenly he stopped and said, curiously, "Hey, what's this?"

His hand had come to rest on her breast and stopped, frozen. He removed it slowly and she saw, through the Lycra suit, what he was referring to. A lump. *The* lump. It was pushing itself out, demanding attention.

She stared at it with uncanny dispassion for a long moment—that instant between sight and recognition. Before the adrenalin hit. Then the panic came—a ring of sweat encircled her neck although she was still chilled from the sea, and her stomach churned. She could see her fear mirrored in Peter's face.

They struggled up from the beach, not speaking, trailing their blanket and towels. The house seemed an interminable distance and the sand, so smooth and sexy a short while ago, was now like a quagmire. In their cramped room she tore at the straps of her bathing suit.

There it was. Her "cyst." But it had grown—how it had grown! How had she not noticed it? Or had she noticed it and repeatedly put it out of her mind, especially on this wonderful vacation? The last time she had examined herself it was a gumball-sized annoyance. Now it was the size of a, well, a walnut at least. It poked out from her breast, arrogantly demanding attention. And it was not, as her gynecologist had suggested, soft or mobile. No, this *thing*, whatever the hell it was, was as hard as a rock and it didn't budge.

"Is that your cyst?" Peter asked dumbly. Normally she would have come back with some wisecrack, but now she just lay there, her hands crossed mummy-style on the bed, freezing but not wanting to move to pull the cover over her.

"I said, is that it? Is that your cyst, Robin?"

"Peter, I think I've got cancer," she finally whispered. The whisper exhausted her, but it also broke the spell, the trance. Suddenly she understood catatonia: she felt like turning into wood and staying that way forever.

"What the hell are you talking about?" he demanded. "You're just a *kid*. You're in perfect health. And besides, you had the damn thing looked at already."

"It's cancer," she repeated.

"Look, I'm sure there's a simple explanation for it," he said, pacing the floor. "The doctor said it was a cyst and it *is* a cyst. I'm sure, Robin. But cysts grow. They fill up with fluid. Women have them all the time, don't they? And besides, hon," he said, sitting on the bed and trying to smile, "you know you've been complaining about your breasts hurting this summer. Your period and all that. This is no different."

"It's different," she said, her chin quivering. She was scared, yet she had to admit, Peter was making sense. Yet somehow this seemed different. Call it intuition. Or fate. It was her mother all over again.

"Hey, listen. Where's my dinner?" Peter said suddenly. "We're not going to sit around here moping all evening, are we? You're going to have a great time your last evening here if I have to *force* you to."

Normally she would have laughed. Peter had a weird sense of humor and, in fact, she could never go with a guy unless he had as strange a sense of humor as herself. But she couldn't laugh. She rolled over, her face in the pillow, and kept repeating something inaudible over and over again.

He sat there, at a total loss for words. He had never seen her like this before—never. Theirs had been a fun relationship. Now this. Then, slowly, the noises stopped.

"You're beautiful when you cry," he whispered.

She rolled over, her face tear-stained. "And you're corny

when you're horny, you bastard." They both started laughing and sobs turned into laughter and laughter into tears.

Robin's gynecologist took one look at her tumor and turned white. He made an appointment for her with Dr. Ruth Snyder, one of the leading breast radiologists in New York City.

Robin took the mammogram and was getting ready to leave when one of the doctors came hurrying out.

"We'd like to do another test," he said, just as she was doing up the last button on her blouse.

"Another test?" she said.

"A sonogram this time."

She tried to remain clam and matter-of-fact, but at that moment, she felt certain they had found breast cancer. I've bought it this time, she said to herself.

The radiologist went on and on about fibroadenomas, about how benign they were, and how four out of five women with lumps only had this kind of harmless tumor. But it was no use: she had seen this happen to her mother. They couldn't fool her.

That evening she had an appointment with Leslie Strong.

It was strange for both of them. She knew him socially. He had been to her apartment. She had served him drinks at Court Street. To have a stranger disrobe in the office was one thing. But for a social acquaintance to disrobe was, if not actually sexual, just a trifle awkward.

Strong had been forewarned by Ruth Snyder. "Pay careful attention to this one," she had said over the phone that afternoon. "It looks terribly suspicious." But when he felt it his heart sank into the pit of his stomach. It was huge by now. He felt under her armpit. The "glands," or nodes, were swollen and hard. While a case of "swollen glands" ordinarily need not be serious, when they are coupled with a breast tumor in the area, they are an ominous sign. It usually means that the cancer has spread beyond its original site. Current thinking on the matter is that cancer cells spread through the blood or the lymph, and the nodes are like little filter stations along the lymph system. Robin's enlarged nodes probably meant that they had been filtering out cancer cells, trying to stop them from entering the rest of the body. With this size tumor, however, and this degree of node involvement, there was little chance they had succeeded.

Cancer patients are placed in one of four categories upon diagnosis. Stage one is a tumor less than two centimeters in diameter with no lymph node involvement. Stage two is a tumor two to five centimeters, with or without positive lymph nodes. Stage three is a tumor greater than five centimeters in size, with positive axillary, or armpit, nodes, but no distant metastases to the bones, liver, lungs, or brain. And stage four is any size tumor with distant metastases already present. If this was malignant then she was already stage three. He couldn't believe this, looking at Robin, this cheerful, funny girl opposite him.

Nor could he tell her this. Not just yet. Not until he was sure.

"Bad news, eh?" she said, watching his face nervously.

"Robin, we're going to have to do a biopsy *but fast,*" he said. "This thing should have come out months and months ago. What the hell happened here? Why did you let it go this long?"

"My gynecologist told me not to worry about it," she said, her voice growing a bit shrill and defensive. "He said I should watch it. So I watched it . . . grow and grow and grow. No, actually, I forgot about it until this summer on the beach. That's when I called you," she said. "I should have come to you in the first place, but I trusted him." She could hardly get the words out, she felt so awful.

"He told you to *watch* this?" Strong practically yelled. "To *watch* it? To watch it do *what?*" He was furious, and his anger focused on her well-known gynecologist.

"Is it cancer?" she asked. "Tell me."

"I can't tell," he said. It was not quite a lie—technically he wouldn't know until the operation. But everything about it screamed out malignancy.

"Four out of five of these turn out . . ."

". . . four out of five are benign. Fibro-whatevers. I know that speech, Leslie, I heard it once already today."

They both laughed, but he wouldn't give in. There was no use in alarming her. The most important thing was to get her into Beth Israel and do an excisional biopsy on this. Then they'd know for sure.

"And what if it is cancer, Leslie?"

"Well, if it is cancer," he said, talking a bit too loud, because of his own agitation, "you'll have a number of alternatives. Such as a modified mastectomy, or possibly radiation therapy. Plus chemotherapy if it turns out to have spread." He tried to make his voice as neutral as possible, not to alarm her. Sometimes these initial conversations were too much for the patients and they ran away from the problem altogether, losing a few more precious months.

"You won't believe me when I tell you that I knew this was coming. My life just parallels my mother's in every respect."

"Well, statistically . . ."

"The hell with statistics. I'm not talking about statistics, Leslie. I'm talking about . . ."

". . . fate?"

"I don't know what I'm talking about," she said, laughing that infectious laugh of hers. "All I know is, life sucks. I knew this would happen. I just didn't think it would happen quite so fast."

When Robin was gone, Strong got her gynecologist on the phone.

"What can I do for you?" asked the doctor, who had a very busy Upper East Side practice.

"Doctor, this is Leslie Strong."

They exchanged pleasantries and the OB-GYN asked casually about some other patients he had sent to Strong in the past. Finally Strong said: "I'd like to talk to you about one of your recent patients, Robin Mack."

There was silence on the other end. "What about her?" the other doctor asked cautiously.

"This woman appears to have a very advanced growth, which is probably going to turn out to be CA upon biopsy."

"I'm very sorry to hear that," said the gynecologist. "She's a nice girl."

"A nice girl?" Strong said, trying with little success to keep the anger out of his voice. "Is it true that you told her you'd *watch* this tumor when you found it earlier this year?"

"What if I did?"

"Doctor," said Strong, breathing hard, "you saw her when she had a small tumor the size of a pea. The nodes probably weren't even involved. Now she has a tumor almost the size of an orange. I can palpate those nodes with no difficulty. Don't you realize what that means?"

"I resent your tone, Doctor," said the gynecologist. "I happen to be a very experienced physician. You can check my credentials with the Board or with the state society or with anyone else. . . ."

Strong knew this was true. In fact, Robin herself and most everyone else swore by him and to all appearances he was a fine gynecologist. The trouble was that he was not a breast specialist. Some of the gynecologists he dealt with had little specialized knowledge of breast disease and the way to work up properly a patient with breast problems. The really smart ones realized this and passed all their breast-disease cases over to breast surgeons, who, for a variety of historical reasons, were the only breast specialists around. This man hadn't realized this quite yet.

"I'm not questioning your credentials," said Strong. "I know your excellent reputation. But don't *you* realize that you can't *watch* a tumor grow? If it's a tumor it *will* grow, and once it has spread beyond the original site . . ." Strong sighed audibly, in exasperation, ". . . the woman's chances are reduced markedly. Dramatically. We can cure localized cancers eighty percent of the time—or at least give the woman five disease-free years. But after it is spread, those odds go down something terrible."

There was silence. "Strong, I feel very sorry about this, but I did the best I could for this patient. I hope you can do better," and he hung up. Strong cringed inside. It was a speech he had heard before, delivered with one eye on the medical book, the other on the law book. Everyone these days, it seemed, was running scared of malpractice suits. Strong realized that this kind of conversation meant that this OB-GYN would probably never send him a referral again. And breast surgeons in private practice like himself *lived* by referrals from gynecologists and other specialists. If the word gets around that you're a troublemaker, *no one* will send you patients. You're simply out of business, unable to help anyone in any way. It was truly a dilemma, and he didn't know the answer. No one knew the answer. But that didn't help poor Robin Mack, who might wake up next Wednesday with some very bad news indeed.

And indeed, Robin's news turned out to be bad, very bad. Just as Strong suspected, her biopsy, performed at Beth Israel, was positive. Considering the fact that her mother had died of breast cancer, the prognosis was, as they said, guarded. They would do the best they could, he explained to her, but there were no guarantees.

After she got over the initial shock, Robin was surprisingly calm. She seemed almost fatalistic: if it had happened to her mother, she felt, then sooner or later it was bound to happen to her as well.

After her biopsy Strong sent Robin to see Dr. Myron Nobler, a radiologist affiliated with the Breast Health Program.

"Dr. Strong wants me to talk to you about your alternatives," said Nobler, as they sat in his Upper East Side office.

"First of all, you have the surgical alternative. You can have a traditional mastectomy—a modified radical. This is a very complete operation. Strong would remove the breast and the lymph nodes. If your bone, brain, and liver scans are all negative, Robin, he will then have removed all visible traces of the tumor."

"What's wrong with that?" she asked.

"Nothing," said Nobler. "But you should be aware that there is an alternative. Instead of removing the whole breast, Strong could only remove the tumor and a quarter of the breast around the tumor. This is called a quadrantectomy. He would also remove the lymph nodes. We could then follow this up with a course of radiation therapy. We generally use Cobalt-sixty teletherapy to the breast and the adjoining lymph-node regions."

"How much radiation is involved?" asked Robin.

"Sometimes we deliver a tumor dose of five thousand rads, delivered in two-hundred-rad increments, for a total of twenty-five treatments over a period of approximately six weeks."

The numbers overwhelmed her. In fact, she was hardly listening. All she heard was the number: 5000 rads. She remembered that her mammogram had been less than half a rad. This man was talking about giving her a dose of 10,000 times that!

And she had been afraid of the possible ill effects of the mammogram.

"Following this," said Nobler, unaware of the anxiety within her, "we deliver a booster dose of radiation to the scar and the tumor bed either by means of an interstitial Iridium-one-ninety-two seed implant, or by electron-beam therapy generated by our eighteen-megavolt linear accelerator."

Robin nodded. The man himself seemed very nice, but she just couldn't relate to all the technological jargon. She felt like she was becoming part of the space program. Some people might feel comforted by the thought of all these wonderful secret beams, but to her it was simply alien and frightening.

"Are you following?" asked Nobler.

"I think so," said Robin. "Basically, my choice is between having it all off now, and living without a breast, or having just a portion of it off, and following this up with some massive doses of radiation."

"You could put it that way," said Nobler, smiling. "Actually it's a bit more complicated than all that."

"But basically you're saying that the more sparing procedure is just as good as the more radical procedure."

"You're putting words in my mouth," said Nobler. "There are some advantages to the more sparing procedure. But, of course, since breast cancer is probably present in a number of locations within the affected breast, it would have to be watched *very* carefully after the sparing procedure. But the choice is yours.

"The point is that you *do* have a choice," he added.

Walking up First Avenue, toward her home, Robin pondered what Nobler had told her. Logically she felt she had nothing to lose from the more sparing procedure and much to gain. Of course, the cancer might always come back to the three-quarters of the breast that were not removed. In that case she could have a mastectomy to remove it all. That would be a rational way of dealing with the problem, she supposed.

But another part of her mind responded in a more emotional way. Get rid of it, this part said. It's bad, rotten. Cut it away! She knew that every time she took a shower, every time Peter touched her there, in the back of her mind she would be waiting for that sickening surprise of discovery.

But do you sacrifice a breast because of such emotional concerns? Wasn't she just being hysterical? Once she did it she couldn't change her mind again. On the other hand . . .

Her thoughts went around in a dizzying spiral like this all week. For a while she hated Leslie Strong and his Breast Health Program. Why didn't she just go somewhere where the doctors would decide for her, where they would just tell her what time of day to show up? Who the hell needs choices, anyway? How could she make a choice like this? But then she realized that someone had to make a choice whenever real alternatives existed. And, after all, it was her body. For thousands of years doctors—almost always males—had made these kinds of choices for women. Now she would have to make the choice for herself.

The day before she went to see Dr. Strong she knew what that choice would be. The quadrantectomy, with its node dissection and radiotherapy, impressed her as modern and innovative. But she still picked the more traditional modified radical mastectomy. She would rather live without the breast than live with additional fears and anxieties, whether they were real or not. She just couldn't stand the uncertainty of knowing that the cancer might return to the unremoved breast.

While the organ scans were all negative for cancer, she still worried that the tumor cells had slipped past the lymph nodes and settled somewhere else in her body. She was irritated with Strong, because he wouldn't give her a definitive answer about this. "You mean to tell me you can't tell if it's in the rest of me?"

"Not really. At the present time medicine is still lacking the tools to tell in every case if cancer has spread beyond the original site. Your scans are all negative, and so we know there is no visible tumor in your brain, bones, liver, or lungs. But micrometastases might be there and we still wouldn't know. In fact, some people consider breast cancer to be a systemic disease from the outset. But at the present time we have to go by what the lymph nodes tell us, and in your case they are flashing a warning signal. That is why chemotherapy is so important, since it might wipe out those small colonies of cells we cannot even see."

"What about that blood test they gave me? I think they call it CEA?"

"Carcino-embryonic antigen," said Strong. "That's the

kind of chemical test we're looking for, but it's still far from perfect. We use it as an indicator of how much cancer is in the body. For instance, we take a CEA reading before the operation. This usually returns to normal after the operation. We will then follow the CEA level throughout your recovery. If the CEA starts to rise it might be an early marker of recurrent disease. Dr. Vogel will take these tests, but I'll be in constant touch with him. But I can't urge you strongly enough to follow through with the chemotherapy, no matter what happens, Robin."

When Strong left, Robin sat in a chair by the window of her room at Beth Israel. Outside the window she could see teenagers streaming out of nearby Stuyvesant High School. She was too high up to hear them, but she could see from their body movements that they were happy and carefree. The way they threw their heads back, or scooted around on the sidewalk, showed that they were still spontaneous and joyful. She felt an indescribable warmth toward them, and tears welled up in her eyes.

It had been such a short time before that she had been as free. Everyone had said so: it was remarkable how youthful she remained. Yet in one crazy moment all that had changed. All she thought about now, all she talked about, was her disease. It dominated all conversations, occupied her mind, and pared her sleeping time at both ends.

Where would it end, she wondered. Like her mother? She wouldn't let it. She had learned from her mother's experience. The innocent child had to grow up sometime. And this, she supposed, was the most important struggle she would ever engage in. She had never liked fighting, but she would have to learn to fight. For this time she was fighting for life itself.

Dr. Strong

Although Strong had gotten many fine doctors to sign up with the Breast Health Program, he had failed to interest any large institutions in the idea. But just when he was feeling the lowest about the prospects of the BHP, he got an encouraging call from Dorothy Wayner.

"Leslie," she said excitedly. "I think I've made a really good contact for you. Dr. Carl Forman wants to meet you."

"The name's familiar," said Strong.

"He's the director of the Eastern Women's Center. It's at fourteen East Sixtieth Street in Manhattan. They've got branches in other cities, as well. And they see thousands of women yearly. Forman's interested in the Breast Health Program."

The Eastern Women's Center was located right off Fifth Avenue. Dr. Forman was a psychiatrist who had started the Eastern Women's Center because he wanted to provide a place where women could get comprehensive treatment. The chief gynecologist at the center turned out to be an acquaintance of Strong's, Dr. Thomas D. Kerenyi.

"We see forty thousand women a year, Dr. Strong," Dr. Forman began when they were seated in his office. "We provide many different health services for women. But after speaking to Dorothy Wayner I realized that there's a big omission in our program. We don't provide comprehensive breast care."

"Few centers do," said Strong.

"Of course, when women come in for examination their breasts are examined by the gynecologist. But we want to do more than that. We want to start a program where these women will become really educated about their breasts and about good preventive care. How would you like to join up with us?"

"What do you have in mind?" asked Strong.

"Well, for starters, Dorothy sent over a copy of your Breast Health Program *Bulletin*. I like it. It's simply written but quite informative. We would like to take bundles of it and put it in our offices, to give it to all the women who come in. That alone could do a lot of good."

"No problem," said Strong. He was delighted.

"Then we'd like to have an arrangement where you present lectures, show films, arrange demonstrations, right here at the Eastern Women's Center. There's a tremendous hunger for good, reliable information, and I think you're just the person to deliver it."

"Fine," said Strong.

"And finally, Strong, we'd like you to do the breast examinations for our women. Right here on the premises. Let's say you'd come in one day a week, examine the women whom the other doctors have found with suspicious symptoms."

"Who's doing that now?"

"As it presently stands, we're referring them back to their personal physicians. But you and I know that many women do not have personal physicians. And of those who do, many of those are not in touch with top-rate breast specialists. In any case, it results in a considerable delay in getting professional help. But with you on the premises on a certain specified day, we could give them an appointment and make sure they show up."

Strong was beaming. He didn't want to look *too* eager, but he just couldn't help himself.

"So what do you say, Strong? Will you come on board? I think we could work very well together. There could be a kind of synergy between the Eastern Women's Center and the Breast Health Program. Each will help the other grow."

"You've got a deal," said Strong enthusiastically. "When do we begin?"

Virginia

It was Thursday evening. Virginia Gipe battled her way up the hill from her office, fighting the biting wind coming off the East River. It was a damp and foggy evening, unusual for summer, and she closed her jacket closer around her neck. The collar felt comforting and warm, if a bit threadbare. She gave a cheerful hello to a group of Watchtower printers also leaving work late, and hurried into the lobby of the Towers.

It was past six o'clock. She had stayed later, working on a computer printout that just had to be done before Monday. No one else in the office could do the job as quickly as she, and so it was a pleasure to undertake the extra work. But she also needed to shower and to eat before the dining room closed. On Thursday nights she and Fred had an appointment at the Theocratic Ministers Hall at eight o'clock. She did not intend to be late. She was never late. Fred was already in their room and was almost finished getting dressed.

"Where were you?" he asked, his blue eyes stern but not unfriendly.

"I'm sorry, Fred," she said. "But I just had to work overtime on that computer printout for the Sierra Leone Missionaries. Without it, their work will be set back, and Brother Joseph is flying over there next Monday."

"Then you did the right thing," said Fred. "Sometimes I am too quick to pass judgments. Like Abraham and Sarah, a husband can often learn from his wife," he said, smiling.

She kissed him on the cheek. "I have to shower, though, before we can go."

"That's all right," said Fred. "We can miss supper tonight. It is no great sacrifice for a Christian."

"That's true," said Virginia, but her heart sank. She was very hungry and had, in fact, skipped lunch because the computer printer had jammed. Maybe I should say something, she thought. After all, the Lord doesn't want us to get sick. But, no, Fred is quite right: if we sit down in the dining room to a supper, we'll never get out to Kew Gardens in time. And what an example we'd set for the students in the Kingdom Hall. Then, if they become missionaries, they will follow our bad example, and so on down the line.

"Perhaps we could pick up something on the way," she said tentatively. She didn't mean to contradict him, of course—after all, God, in Ephesians, taught us that a woman must be in subjection to her husband. But her stomach was growling in involuntary disobedience.

"Perhaps," he said slowly. Virginia knew what he was thinking. First of all, he did not like to eat out. It smacked of pleasure-seeking, of needless and pointless entertainment for its own sake. Second, the quality of the food one got outside was uncertain. And, finally there was the question of money. As volunteers, they were not paid for their hard labor at "Bethel," the name Jehovah's Witnesses gave to their World Headquarters in downtown Brooklyn. Each of them got a thirty-dollar monthly allowance. What would happen if they spent their little money on coffee, doughnuts, and pizza? It would quickly disappear. And then what would happen if they got sick or had some other emergency?

"No, I guess you're right," said Virginia. "It's not so important. I can wait." She felt good about her decision. It was important to act like a true Christian woman, not a hypocrite.

She carefully removed her clothes and draped them over the chair. It was an ornate chair that surprised visitors to their "apartment," a small room in what had once been the Towers Hotel. She had brought a number of things from home as reminders—her grandmother's blond Victrola case was her favorite—but the rest had been sold when they moved to New York three years ago. In a way, the spirit of their former home was still present in this miniature version.

Fred turned away as she disrobed. He busied himself unfolding the Murphy bed he had built into the wall. It was truly ingenious. Fred was descended from four generations of Bavarian and German-American woodworkers, and although he had gone into graphic arts as his life work, he was still so good with his hands.

Virginia showered carefully, stretching her neck under the hot water to relieve the tension of the day. She felt like she needed a vacation. The pace of life in New York was so unbelievably fast. How could people stand it, it was so *inhuman.* Even the way they spoke was abnormal, like a long-playing phonograph record played at 78 rpm. It was almost comical to a person like her from the South. Of course, she realized that she was in a strange territory, almost another country altogether, and would have to adapt herself to the local customs just as the brothers and sisters in Africa or Asia often did. Yet she looked forward to a week coming up at home in Owensboro, Kentucky. It would be so wonderful, so relaxing. She couldn't wait to hear English spoken normally again!

She soaped herself up, but went lightly over her breast area. As usual, she felt a bit guilty. Several years ago—when she was still Mrs. Gipe, the suburban housewife of Owensboro—she had had a lump in her breast. Her doctor, an old family practitioner, had carefully and gently examined her. "I wouldn't be too alarmed at this, Virginia. It's common enough for a woman in her forties to get a little lump now and then. Why don't you just wait until your next monthly occurrence and then come back and see me." He gave her a bottle of medicine, which she took a teaspoon of every day. And the lump did go away. It was nothing.

Fred, however, was always after her to examine herself. "Please, Virginia," he'd say, "we need you to be *well* to help carry out Jehovah's plan for us. Doesn't the Bible tell us," he added, his face calm and strong, "in Second Corinthians, to cleanse ourselves of every defilement of flesh and spirit? Don't you agree this means to keep our bodies in a healthy condition?"

He was right, of course, but she was weak. Fear kept her from touching herself there, much less practicing any regular kind of breast self-examination. It was wrong, but it was just a small self-indulgence of hers.

She emerged from the bath feeling calmer and more refreshed, and ready for her evening duties. They had meetings every night except Fridays now. There was Kingdom Hall—what other people called "church services"—at least twice a week. There was their Bible Study Group, as well as the joyful responsibility to carry Jehovah's message door to door in Rego Park, Queens. But of all her work she enjoyed these Thursday nights the best. For this was Theocratic Ministers night. The enthusiasm of these young ministers, many of whom were going to carry the news of Jehovah's Kingdom to strange foreign shores, was a marvel to behold. They were so loving, so filled with enthusiasm and fervor. Such an atmosphere provoked her to greater sacrifices.

Virginia reached for a pair of shoes in the top of the shoe rack that hung from the door of their only closet. Despite her voluntary poverty, she had not lost her good taste in clothes. She still wore stockings every day and her diamond engagement ring and white gold wedding band. She had even been secretly flattered when a non-Witness delivery man had whispered to her one day, "You know, you're one classy dame!" Of course she had turned away, because the Bible was very clear, in the story of David and Bathsheba, that even an uncontrolled glance can prove fatal. But, at forty-nine, she was proud of her youthful looks and attractive form. She intended to stay so, as long as possible, to remain attractive for Fred, as a wife should be, and to have her looks be an asset to the church.

As she reached up, her hand brushed against her side and she felt something. It was not anything big, and she continued to remove the pair of beige shoes that matched the beige suit she had found in a Brooklyn Heights thrift shop for ten dollars. She sat down on the edge of the bathtub to pull on her stockings, but she sensed that something was out of order.

There was no time to waste, of course, but she tentatively reached up again and laid her hand gingerly on her breast. Nothing. She moved her hand up higher, her fingertips practically into her armpit, and then her heart froze. For there beneath the skin she definitely *felt something.* She pulled her hand away, and told herself, hurry up, Virginia. Keep this up and we'll be late for sure.

Fred was humming in the other room. That usually meant he was becoming impatient. No, I must find out if this is something real, or if I imagined it. She put her hand on the area more definitively, and focused in with her sensitive fingers. Oh my God! There is something! She could move it around, like rolling a little pea between her fingers. She let her hand drop. A long moment went by and she imagined that her face must be ashen. Her throat suddenly felt dry as the Sinai.

"Fred," she yelled, her voice quaking. "Could you please come here for a minute?"

Fred stepped across the small room and stood in the doorway of the bathroom.

"What is it?" he asked, a bit alarmed at her tone of voice. "What's wrong?"

Virginia wrapped a large towel around her nakedness. She had never felt quite right being looked at by a man in this way, not even her own husband of eighteen years. "Do you think . . . this is something?" she asked. She directed his hand to the spot she had found.

Fred rubbed his finger back and forth over it.

"Am I imagining it? Or . . ."

"No, there's definitely something there," he said, after deliberating for a moment. "Does it hurt you?"

"No, I can't say that it does," she said, encouraged by this fact. "I just wanted to make sure I wasn't imagining it."

Fred appeared deep in thought, his jaw cradled in his strong hand: he squeezed his mouth together pensively.

"I know that, whatever happens, the Lord will provide. But perhaps it would be best for you to go see Dr. Corey in the morning," he added.

Virginia nodded. Dr. Corey was a young woman, a sister, who operated the clinic here at Bethel. She would never criticize a sister, of course, but in her mind she wondered if Dr. Corey was experienced enough to deal with this. But what am I thinking, of course she is. They wouldn't let her be a doctor at Bethel if she weren't. All the top directors use her as well. And besides, this is just a false alarm, just like the other time.

As they were walking to the subway—at double-time because they were now very possibly going to be late—Virginia said, "Fred, you don't think this is going to turn out to be—something?"

"Of course not," said Fred reassuringly. "But, Virginia, if the Lord chooses to test us in this way, I'm sure we're ready for it. And look at Job. He had everything taken away, but then it was restored to him twofold. There's a lesson in that."

"Yes, there is," said Virginia, but at the moment she couldn't remember exactly what that lesson was.

On the day after she discovered the lump, Virginia went to see Dr. Corey. The Witnesses maintained a large, modern infirmary on the premises, with a doctor either in attendance or on call at all times. And all such medical treatment was free of charge to the 2300 members of the Bethel community.

"How long ago did you discover this?" asked Dr. Corey. She was a thin woman, new to the faith, and she seemed a bit nervous—or perhaps Virginia was just projecting her own nervousness.

"Just yesterday," she said. "After my bath."

"Do you ordinarily practice breast self-examination?" asked Dr. Corey. It was just a routine question, but to Virginia, at that moment, it sounded accusatory.

Virginia hesitated. "No, I don't. I just found it by accident."

Dr. Corey frowned and Virginia felt suddenly alarmed. "Is this . . . something to be concerned about?"

"How old are you, Sister Virginia?"

"I'm forty-nine," she said.

"Well, I wouldn't have guessed!" said Dr. Corey, and Virginia smiled, appreciating the kind word. She was feeling much older these days, and, in fact, when she woke up that morning, she was alarmed at how "old-ladyish" her face looked, almost as if she were turning into her own mother before her very eyes. One could become depressed about such things, if one didn't believe that Jehovah would restore the Righteous to their perfect, youthful selves on Judgment Day.

"At your age *any* lump is a concern," said Dr. Corey. "But most often these things are related to your menses. Therefore,

I'd like to wait a month till your next menses and then examine you again."

"Is it all right for Brother Fred and me to go down to Kentucky?" she asked in her slow drawl.

"And I don't see why not," said Dr. Corey. "Just make sure you don't forget to see me upon your return."

Virginia gathered up her office stuff—printed lists of names she had to deliver to the headquarters building. It was reassuring. By the time she returned to work she could forget about the whole thing.

Owensboro was a lovely town of fifty thousand situated on the banks of the meandering Ohio River, in the western part of the state. Even in the midwinter the temperatures here were moderate, the pace of life slow. It was a welcome change from the hustle and bustle of New York City, even if it was just for two weeks.

Virginia had spent her entire life in Owensboro—except for three months spent in Frankfort (Kentucky, she always had to explain, not Germany). She had graduated from the regional high school and then gone to junior college at night for some accounting courses. Then she had taken a job at the Imperial Furniture Company, the largest business in town. The chief of art, advertising, public relations, and community relations at the works was a young fellow named Fred Gipe. Fred was a handsome man, in his mid-thirties when she met him, with pale blue eyes and a gentle manner. But underneath his gentleness she sensed manly strength and determination, as well as a keen intelligence. Although Fred Gipe had never gone to college, he was knowledgeable about many topics, and, most importantly, the Bible. In Owensboro, knowledge of chapter and verse was a very important gauge of a man's mind and character.

Fred Gipe was a widower: it was common knowledge in the town that his wife had died in a Lexington hospital at the age of twenty-five of a subarachnoid hemorrhage. Virginia was never sure what a subarachnoid hemorrhage was, but she was impressed by Fred's calm acceptance of God's will in taking his young and beautiful wife from him and leaving him to raise a five-year-old boy by himself.

They were married soon afterward and theirs had been a

happy marriage. They were both attractive people, with normal human drives. But what attracted her most about Fred was the strength he provided to their marriage, the firm hand in directing their affairs. As a woman, she felt a bit inadequate in dealing with the complexities and difficulties of modern life. She wondered sometimes what she would have done if she had never met Fred.

If people asked her, as they inevitably did, how she came to be one of Jehovah's Witnesses, she would tell them "one of her fellow employees" taught her the truth about God's Kingdom. Actually, that "fellow employee" was none other than Fred. She didn't like the looks she sometimes got when she admitted that: ah ha, you fell in love with this handsome widower and *that's* why you converted. The knowing looks. That was not exactly why, however. She had been born and raised a Baptist, but had never felt that her native-born religion adequately lived up to the word of the Scriptures. To her, there was never any question that Scripture was indeed the literal word of God, but many nominal Christians treated God's word very lightly indeed. They had their Sunday morals and their weekday morals, just as they had their Sunday clothes and their workaday clothing. This, to her, was the sickening hypocrisy of Pharisees, not Christian rectitude. You might as well abandon religion altogether and have yourself a fling than hold to a two-faced creed.

Fred agreed with her but had shown her the way. There was only *one* Church on earth, he explained, that prepared the way for God's coming and the establishment of paradise on earth. So many things she had been taught from the Bible turned out to be misinterpreted or misunderstood.

"God is quite explicit that we must worship Him in His name," said Fred, and he provided her with the appropriate Biblical citation. "As his name is Jehovah, we must call him by that name. Now, if I speak of myself as a follower of Jehovah, what religion would you associate me with?" he asked didactically.

"Jehovah's Witnesses?" she had offered.

"Precisely. The one true form of Christianity, which is not afraid to speak the name of the Lord it worships."

Virginia had had scant contact with the Witnesses before this—once or twice they had been politely turned away when they came to her father's door. But she was enraptured with her new husband and with his beliefs. She was herself baptized in a stirring ceremony and accepted into the Church in 1969.

Virginia sat in the kitchen of the old house where she was born and told her mother, as casually as she could manage, that she had found "a little something" in her breast.

"Well, that's nothing to worry about," said her mother. "Plenty of women have those sorts of things all the time. All of this radio and TV" (she said it like she was fishing for a new word) "scare you half to death about this and that. But I'm sure it'll turn out to be nothing."

Virginia felt so good to be back in the calico-cheerful kitchen, redolent of nutmeg, cinnamon, and allspice, talking to her dear mother. It was just like old times. They were truly fortunate. She had lived to see her parents grow into old age. They were well-secured, owned their own house, and Father had a decent enough pension from the factory. All was well. Of course, sometimes they quarreled—like when Fred and she refused to celebrate Christmas, have a tree, or exchange presents.

"The shepherds were out in the fields when Jesus was born," said Fred, vehemently overriding her father's objections. "That shows that it could not have been the rainy season of winter. Besides, as the *Encyclopedia Brittanica* itself says, December twenty-fifth was a pagan holiday." Virginia's father sucked on his pipe and listened. Fred was a nice fellow and all, but Dad went on decorating his Christmas tree and giving out little presents to all the kids in the neighborhood. And despite the fact that she knew Fred was right theologically, it still cheered her heart to come home late at night in Owensboro and see the green and red lights, the presents in gold and silver foil heaped up under the tree, and the red cheeks of the Church carolers.

Back in New York, however, the news was not good. Virginia went to see Dr. Corey soon after her next period. As she knew from gingerly feeling herself, the lump was still there, high up on her breast. If anything, she imagined it was now even a bit larger. Fred said it was the size of a pencil eraser. That sounded about right, but the image somehow stayed with her and haunted her. What was this rubbery thing doing in her body? Dr. Corey suggested she see Dr. Dixon, a Witness surgeon. "Virginia," he said kindly, "this sort of thing can upset a woman. Let's go in and take it out."

Even before she spoke to him she had made the decision that she wanted it out. She couldn't stand the uncertainty of living this way. It was impossible to get any work done. She found her thoughts wandering to that little "pencil eraser," and her hand floated up to her breast involuntarily. What good could she do for Jehovah like this? The Witnesses were so well organized at their Brooklyn headquarters that it was no trouble for Dr. Dixon to remove the tiny growth himself in the infirmary under a local anesthetic. He sewed her up with a few stitches and then the specimen was packed in ice and sent out for examination by a pathologist.

The next day Virginia was back in his office. A young nurse was arranging instruments on a tray. "Would you leave us for a moment?" the doctor asked her as soon as Virginia entered.

From that moment she *knew* that the news was not going to be good.

"Virginia," he said slowly, looking away for a moment. "I hate to tell you this more than anything in the world, but there's cancer cells in that specimen I took out yesterday." He paused. "It's definitely malignant."

Virginia sat with her mouth open. She was in shock. I'm not hearing what I'm hearing, she told herself. This is impossible. A month of reassurances—from Fred, her mother, her friends, and, most of all, herself—had really convinced her that this little thing was nothing. It would be just like last time.

Virginia broke out into a cold sweat. She didn't cry, but her eyes watered up, and she felt an overwhelming desire to escape from the stuffy offices into the outdoors.

"Virginia, you're going to need further surgery, major surgery," Dixon said carefully. "I could do it in a local hospital, of course, but I really want you to have the best for this. I'm going to call this afternoon, if it's all right with you and your husband, and make an appointment for you to see Dr. Leslie Strong. For my money, Strong is the best in the business."

Virginia hardly heard a thing. She felt like she couldn't breathe until she heard the infirmary door shut behind her and felt the cool breeze on her face. It felt so good, so refreshing. No, this couldn't be. Couldn't be. Cancer! But how? And why? No one in her family had ever had cancer. They were healthy. *She* was healthy, and yet she had cancer. It made no sense.

She pushed herself up the hill, heading absentmindedly toward Fred's office. Fred worked in one of the thirteen huge buildings that make up the headquarters. People passed her and said hello, calling her by name. She knew many of the brothers and sisters at Bethel by name but this time she ignored them, or rather, didn't even hear them. Tears welled up in her eyes, but she did not break down. She pushed on, as against some vast opposing tide of air that had suddenly risen up to oppose her. And in her mind was one thing: she would have to go in for major surgery. Major surgery meant cutting deep and relentlessly. And cutting meant blood, not the small amount Dr. Dixon had caused with his biopsy, but possibly a serious loss.

Only a Jehovah's Witness, in her hour of darkness, can know what this means. For Witnesses believe that it is absolutely forbidden to receive blood transfusions. They absolve their doctors before hand of any responsibility for not giving such transfusions, and even then few doctors outside the creed will treat them. The question of blood transfusions was a dividing line between the Witnesses and not just the medical profession but practically the rest of humanity. And, therefore, each operation became a test of faith, a trial by scalpel, probing the depth of one's belief, as well as one's body.

Would she stand up to this trial? What would happen if this Dr. Strong was not as careful as Dr. Dixon believed. He was not a Witness, although he must be a brother in spirit to undertake this operation at all. But what if he got careless, and his knife slipped? In her mind's eye she pictured the whole scenario and felt a dark terror, like an approaching thunder cloud. She would die, as she had heard others whispered about: pint after pint pouring out onto the operating table, soaking the draped garments, with the doctors unable to staunch the flow or to give the necessary replacement.

And why was this? She knew, of course. She had given out copies of their pamphlet "Jehovah's Witnesses and the Question of Blood" to many unbelievers and studied it in Bible classes. Yet, strangely, at the moment, she couldn't remember what the reason was, besides the fact that it was in the Bible. All she could think of was that she had cancer and was going to die, either from the disease itself or, before that, on the operating table.

Fred! Fred would know! She battled her way up the hill and arrived, panting, at the door of his office.

A husband's duty, Fred firmly believed, was to provide leadership in the family. Man was created to provide such leadership. For a family to be without leadership, or what the Witnesses called "headship," would be like driving a car without a steering wheel. But headship meant more than just giving orders (although the Bible gave him the authority to do that when necessary). It meant being responsible and caring, the way Jesus cared for all humanity.

All this came to him, with sickening force, as he sat at his desk and saw Virginia standing in the doorway of his office. He could tell from the terrible look on her face and the tears that were just now bursting forth that the news was bad.

The strange thing, and the disturbing thing, was that he had not been there when she needed him most. All their lives together, for almost twenty years, they had been not just husband and wife, but best friends. They always said that, and they meant it. He used to go with her to the doctor for even minor things. Yet for some reason he could not fathom, but which greatly bothered him, he had not been there when she really needed him.

"Well, it's bad news," she blurted out, her voice cracking.

"Cancer?" he asked.

She nodded. "Dr. Dixon said he wants to talk to you, Fred."

He came around the desk, where he was working on the design of the next *Watchtower* cover, and put his arm around her. She sobbed bitterly now, uncontrollably.

"I'm sorry, Virginia. I should have been there."

"Don't be silly, you had no way—"

"I can't understand my stupidity. Perhaps I had a premonition and was afraid? But no, I just took it too lightly. I thought it was something insignificant. We convinced ourselves it was nothing. And now this!"

She nodded in agreement, and, in the depth of her own anguish, she suddenly felt terribly sorry for her husband. He had lost one wife. Would he now lose another?

"Let us not be alarmist about this," he said, regaining his composure. "I rather this would be me," he said. "But this is the real world. This is the actual situation. We know very little about the whole topic. We've got to get the true picture."

"But where do we begin?" Virginia asked.

Fred's mind automatically reached for an appropriate Biblical quotation. After all, the Bible is a *practical* book—he firmly believed that—and had advice on every sort of question. Yet somehow, for some reason, he too drew a blank. Timothy? Acts? Leviticus? He sat there with his mouth ready to speak, but no words came out. He just shook his head back and forth slowly in bewilderment.

Dr. Dixon made the appointment for Virginia with Dr. Strong for the following Tuesday.

Virginia was in a state of panic all week. She had tried to go to work every day. One time, as she was talking to her supervisor, Harry Billard, about the best way to process Regular Pioneer applications, she just broke down and started sobbing uncontrollably. She ran from the office. Later Harry sent her a note that read simply, "For the eyes of Jehovah are upon the righteous and his ears are toward their supplication." 1 Peter 3:12. He also referred her to 2 Corinthians 4:7–18. Virginia felt the Christian love pouring out of him and everyone in the office who had learned of her problem. She got out her Bible, read the passages, and cried, this time with happiness. "So encouraging to me," she wrote next to the passage, and she jotted in the name "Harry" so she would always remember this moment, and so that she could better console some other poor soul in the future.

And naturally she prayed. She prayed to Jehovah for direction, for guidance. "Lord, make me able to cope with this terrible problem. Help me to be a mature Christian. Don't let me act in a hopeless fashion and be a bad example to others. Above all, help me to be calm."

In a wild moment, she thought she might pray to God to remove the problem altogether. After all, maybe Dr. Dixon was wrong. He could call her up and say (a bit sheepishly!), Look, we made a mistake. A human error. Not malignant . . . But no. That would be a miracle, and she knew that the age of miracles had passed, that God had performed miracles at the time of

Jesus in order to impress people with the truth of Christ's mission; since that was no longer necessary, miracles were now impossible.

Yet she was troubled. She knew of many people back home in Owensboro who not only believed in faith healing, but claimed that such cures were a common, practically everyday occurrence. Could they all be wrong? Or would God listen to the heartfelt prayers of a woman afraid of death? These were disturbing thoughts, heresy for a Witness, but in the end she concluded she was just being childish in thinking this way. She would have to face the music. Her cancer was a fact, and God could not, or rather would not, intervene. He might intervene in her heart to make her stronger, though.

In the week before they went to see Dr. Strong, they read everything they could get their hands on about breast cancer. Fred spoke to several people whose wives had undergone various kinds of procedures. One of them had had just a partial mastectomy. But the cancer came back repeatedly—seven times, in fact—and she eventually had to have the whole breast removed.

Their first meeting with Dr. Strong was tense and, for Virginia, a bit traumatic.

Strong was nervous. Dealing with the Jehovah's Witnesses was risky business. First of all, their religious beliefs were so unusual that he felt it was easy to step on their toes, to say or do the wrong thing. Many of them came from out of town and seemed thoroughly discombobulated by big city life. Then there was the question of blood. They refused transfusions. He didn't understand all the reasons for this, but nothing he had heard convinced him this was anything more than a religious crotchet. But naturally, as a surgeon it made him nervous. Blood transfusions—along with anesthesia and antisepsis—was one of things that made the modern, prolonged operation possible. It was an essential item in the doctor's tool bag. To take it away, banish it from the operating room, was like doing surgery with one hand tied behind your back.

For that reason most surgeons refused to treat Jehovah's Witnesses.

Strong felt otherwise. His goal was to extend the Breast Health Program so that the maximum number of women were receiving adequate care for their breasts, whether they felt a lump or not. While there was a risk in operating on Witnesses, he felt there was a greater risk in *not* treating them—time lost in treating breast disease could be fatal.

In the back of his mind, always, was the nightmare thought that an operation on a Witness could get out of control and the patient could bleed to death. He had actually seen that happen once, when he was a resident at Downstate. It had been a long and difficult operation on an old man with colon cancer. An artery had been severed—such things happened sometimes, despite the best precautions—and the man started to bleed profusely. They were about to give the man an emergency transfusion when the surgeon in charge informed them that the patient was a Jehovah's Witness. He had agreed not to provide a transfusion under any condition, even the threat of imminent death. The hospital had obtained the necessary forms, absolving it of any responsibility. Of course, the operating team fought valiantly to try and staunch the flow of blood, to tie it off or cauterize it. But it was too late. The man had lost too much blood: the sheets were soaked through with it. And, to their horror, he expired on the operating table. It had been one of the worst things Strong had seen as a resident—and one doesn't serve in a hospital like King's County without seeing one's share of horrors.

Mr. Gipe had come prepared with a list of questions. Strong made him ask them one at a time.

"Well, first of all, doctor, how serious is this problem?"

Strong looked at him incredulously. What had Dixon told these people, he wondered.

"This is very serious. Your wife—" He automatically lapsed into talking to Mr. Gipe, clearly in charge, despite his conscious efforts to always address himself to the woman involved. "—is a very sick woman. I know she doesn't *look* very sick. But the position of her cancer, in the upper outer quadrant, makes it very likely that cancer cells have spread to the axillal area—that's the armpit, in plain English."

The Gipes were struggling to take it all in. All Virginia heard was "very sick" and her mind went in on itself.

Fred was writing everything down in a little notebook. Their God was a God of organization. He himself couldn't be less so.

"I see," said Gipe slowly. "And what treatment alternatives do we have?"

"Basically two," said Strong. "I could remove a quarter of the breast. That's called a quadrant resection. This would be followed up by radiation therapy to the affected breast. The other alternative is a modified radical mastectomy. Do you know what that is?"

"I believe I do," said Fred.

"I was asking Mrs. Gipe," Strong said, suddenly realizing that the conversation was being carried out for her in proxy, as it were.

"Please tell me," said Virginia, and Strong could tell that despite her religious strictures, this was a strong-willed woman with a mind of her own.

"In the modified radical, we remove the breast as well as the lymph nodes in the armpit, but we preserve the muscles of the chest wall. We leave enough of the skin to be able to do future reconstructive surgery. Do you understand?"

"I think so," said Virginia slowly.

"You think so," said Strong, a bit sarcastically. He had had a long day. "What am I doing wrong? What am I not making clear?" He could see the growing distress on Mrs. Gipe's face. "I want this to be totally clear so you can make a decision. Tell me. Speak." He feared he wasn't getting through to Virginia, and that ultimately the decision would be made for her by her husband or perhaps by some board of elders somewhere.

Virginia, for her part, was distressed by what she regarded as his badgering, and found herself on the verge of tears. Why did he speak like this to her? He was so . . . Yankee! In Owensboro doctors like her old G.P. were so slow and easygoing and soft-spoken, just like the rest of the people. They took their time to explain and a little extra time to inquire about the family's health. But up here everyone seemed so cold and impersonal, at least those she met outside the faith.

She was here to do Jehovah's work, but she wondered why the world headquarters had to be located in Brooklyn, of all places, and not in Tennessee or Kentucky or the Carolinas or someplace civilized. But it wasn't. And if the Lord had chosen to bring her to this place, it must be for some good purpose. She would try harder to be understanding.

"That doesn't sound like a very 'modified' operation to me," she said finally. "It sounds like I'm still going to lose my breast."

"Good point," said Strong. "You will, if you choose that route."

"What's the advantage to it, then?"

"The advantage is that you won't spend the rest of your life worrying if the cancer will return in that breast. You will have enough to worry about without adding that burden."

"Do we have time to think about it?" she asked.

"Not much," said Strong. "I would like to make an appointment for you to be admitted next week." He whipped out his pocket calendar, stuffed thick with memos, cards, odds and ends. "Next Wednesday I think I can get you in. You'll have until next Tuesday to make your decision."

"I think we can do that," said Fred Gipe slowly.

"Any more questions?" asked Strong. "Please don't be afraid to ask *anything.*"

"I do have one more," said Fred. "What can we expect from this treatment?"

"Well, that depends on what we find upon operating. When I examined your wife just now I felt some enlarged lymph nodes. That probably means the cancer has already spread to the armpit. In that case, the prognosis is not quite as good as if it was localized. She will need chemotherapy for a year after the operation."

"But what are her . . . chances?" asked Fred.

"Her chances should be good if the operation is a success and if she follows up on it with chemotherapy. I can't give you an exact figure without knowing the extent of her disease, and even then it doesn't take into account other factors. Mental and emotional factors, questions of attitude, which can influence the course of illness."

Actually, Strong thought, the odds of surviving more than five years with disseminated disease were *not* very good, but there was no point in driving that home now. His job at the moment was to buy her confidence, build up her fighting spirit for the surgery. And if faith played any part in healing, as many doctors secretly believed, this woman would have a leg up on the problem.

"Now, Dr. Strong, you understand our position on blood transfusions, I take it," said Fred.

"I can't say that I *understand* it," said Strong. "But I do understand that you don't want any. I'm willing to go along with that. I have to warn you, however, that this makes my job more difficult and makes surgery riskier."

"We understand that," said Fred.

Strong wasn't going to say anything contrary. He strongly believed a person's religious beliefs were their own business. But he couldn't resist asking, "Where exactly in the Bible does it say that a man can't have a blood transfusion? I mean, transfusions weren't even *invented* until the twentieth century."

"Of course, it doesn't say anything directly about blood transfusions," said Fred, happy to discuss the subject. "But it has a lot to say about taking blood into the body. You know, when God first granted us humans the right to devour animal flesh, he told Noah, 'Every moving animal that is alive may serve as food for you. Only flesh with its soul—its blood—you must not eat.' And in Leviticus the Lord says that 'the soul of the flesh is in the blood!' " He emphasized each word with his ballpoint pen. "God also told the hunters to pour the blood of animals on the ground because 'the soul of every sort of flesh is in the blood.' I think the case is quite definitive."

"I see," said Strong. He had heard about as much as he wanted to know. The man's thinking was so odd! Strong was used to thinking in scientific and secular terms. For him the question of blood transfusion, as of everything else medical, was simply one of efficacy versus risk. He knew that there were dangers involved in blood transfusion—the transmission of viral disease such as hepatitis being high on the list—but these were overshadowed by the innumerable life-saving benefits. For the Gipes, however, it all came down to "how do I know, the Bible tells me so." It absolutely blew his mind, since, in other respects, the Gipes seemed like normal, happy, and intelligent people. But being a native New Yorker, Strong had grown up among all kinds of people, and learned the rough-and-tumble tolerance that comes from metropolitan life. If that's their bag, so be it. He wouldn't interfere.

"Mrs. Gipe, I will see you next Tuesday. I hope you will have decided on which treatment you want. I'm giving you a list of other breast specialists in the New York area. It's a routine feature of the Breast Health Program to urge patients to seek second, even third opinions before coming to a decision. But remember, whatever anyone tells you, the choice is *yours.*" He shot a meaningful glance over at her husband, who stared back at him without hostility, but without fear.

Virginia decided she would pass this week like every other. But her mind was not on her work. She had listened to Dr. Strong, but the doubts had only grown with knowledge. Fred had taken a hands-off attitude: he would gather information for her, he said, but he felt firmly that the ultimate decision was hers. He was exercising proper headship, she knew, but sometimes she wished he would simply *tell* her what to do. But, despite appearances, that was not Fred's way.

At first glance, the "quadrant resection," as Dr. Strong called it, seemed the proper way to go. After all, she would only lose one quarter of her breast. Radiation therapy did not hurt, she believed, and so why not take the path of least pain and disfigurement?

On the other hand, the mastectomy seemed more thorough. She also didn't like the idea of waking up each morning afraid of a new lump in her breast. And if the modified radical was safer, then logically it should also help extend her life better. But then she wondered how she could live, just half a woman. Was it true, as Strong said, that she could be reconstructed and regain a good appearance? She was no longer young, she knew that, but she was still attractive to her husband. What would happen when she was as flat as a board on one side? Of course, Fred said that he would still love her as much. But she knew that changes come over a man even despite himself. Could a man still be really attracted to a woman who had a big scar down her chest instead of a well-shaped breast? It was her duty to give him pleasure: the Bible, in First Corinthians 7, told her to "render unto her husband his due." Could she still do that in such an altered condition?

Finally, she decided that she would have the modified radical: she must have as many years or months as possible to spread God's word. The "quadrantectomy" seemed too new, too innovative. She'd stick with the tried and true, even though it would mean the loss of her breast.

On Sunday afternoon she went with Fred and other members of her study group to bring the message of God's visible organization to the good people of Kew Gardens, Queens. They had called on a number of houses before, but there had been no answer, or the people were too busy to talk. And so they returned patiently. At one house they found a young man who invited them in.

He was named Barry and he seemed to be around twenty-five years old. He was good-looking—lean and a bit severe, with a sarcastic manner about him. He seemed eager to talk, though, and offered them coffee, which they declined. Virginia did accept a glass of orange juice, just to show she was not being standoffish.

Barry was a medical technician in a hospital. Inevitably the discussion came around to the question of blood.

"I've known a few Witnesses," he said. "In school, for instance, they always seemed a bit wigged out because they didn't salute the flag or celebrate holidays. Not even their own birthdays! We called them the Witlesses," he said, eyeing them for a reaction.

Virginia smiled; she had heard every derogatory term, had had doors slammed in her face, and even once was spat upon —by a devout "Christian," no less! And she was hardly shocked or offended.

"There is a very good scriptural reason for that," said Fred, whipping out his *New World Translation of the Holy Scriptures.*

"I'm sure there is," said Barry. "But I for one do not believe that the Holy Scriptures, as you call them, are the word of God."

Fred seemed ready for this tack: dealing with unbelievers, in fact, was something of his specialty. Virginia was a little thrown off by the young man's self-assurance. Usually she would be unaffected. *It must be all the disturbances I've been through and the agitation in my soul.*

"Who then do you think wrote the Holy Word?"

"The Holy Word," said Barry ironically, "was written by ordinary men just like you and me—or at least just like you. Religious believers. Some of it is quite lovely. Some of it is quite ugly—especially the mass killings and so forth. But it bears all the earmarks of a historical document assembled out of bits and pieces written over many centuries, and passed down with numerous changes and emendations over many more centuries.

All this was proven more than a hundred years ago. To take such a hodgepodge as the 'word of God' just shows that your minds are stuck back in the Middle Ages somewhere. Can't you see that?"

"You're simply wrong," said Fred self-assuredly. "There are actually very few orthographical errors in the Bible. We have a pamphlet on that if you would like to see it." He snapped open his neat, square briefcase and revealed a regular traveling salesman's worth of books, pamphlets, and reprints, all neatly organized. "The Bible is the literal word of God, and the men who wrote it are no more responsible for its contents than a secretary is responsible for the words of her employers."

Barry laughed. "Spare me. And you know what I think the most ridiculous belief of all is? Blood transfusions! That's got to take the cake. We've had a few patients in our hospital who have refused blood transfusions on religious grounds. And I think it's helped shove them over a bit quicker, if you get my meaning."

Virginia felt very uncomfortable with the drift of the conversation.

"There is no proof that anyone has ever died because they failed to get a blood transfusion," said Fred.

"That's hogwash, and you know it," said Barry. "Blood transfusions are a life-saving thing. People die all the time for lack of them. If you were in a war, on the battlefield, you'd sing a different tune."

"Well, we Witnesses do not fight in man's wars. We do not take sides in the battles of Satan, neither those of the Anglo-American entity, nor those of Red China or Communist Russia or any world power. You know the Bible prophesies that there will be seven world powers, and that these seven will further generate an eighth. And this is indeed what has happened. The eighth is, of course, the United Nations."

Barry shook his head slowly. "I'm glad you don't take part in wars. Because I'd hate to be in a war against *you people!* But if you were, I'm sure you would be crying out for blood transfusions fast enough. Start bleeding and you'd change your mind pronto about the whole thing."

"That's not true," said Virginia. She hesitated, not sure if she should say anything. Then she thought, why let pride hold me back? For the sake of God I must open my heart to this brother, who deserves salvation as much as anyone. "As a matter of fact, I am due to go in for surgery next week. And I do not intend to allow any blood transfusions."

Barry seemed somewhat chastened by this, and also a bit embarrassed. "I'm sorry," he mumbled. "But you haven't had surgery yet. You might change your mind."

"Don't worry, brother. I will not change my mind about this. The Bible is quite explicit on this point. And what if I *were* to die? Don't you realize that Armageddon is coming soon? Within the lifetime of those born in 1914. So you see, I'd only be dead a short time before the Resurrection, and then I'd be rejoined with my whole family. And so, which is worse, Barry, to be dead for a short time and then resurrected, or to remain dead for all eternity?"

"I never really thought about it," said Barry, laughing.

"Well, I think we've taken up enough of your time." Fred always knew when to stop. He pulled out one of his pamphlets, "The Question of Blood," with a picture of a doctor explaining the issue to a clean-cut family. It seemed the most appropriate piece of literature. "Please take this as a gift," he said. "I hope it will help you to answer some of the questions that are obviously disturbing you."

"I'm not the one who's disturbed," said Barry.

"Barry," said Virginia. "We'd like to come back after my operation and talk to you. Then we can discuss the question of blood transfusions again. I'd like that very much."

Barry turned the booklet over in his hands and flipped through the stiff pages, shaking his head in disbelief.

"Would that be okay?" she asked. Fred had his pen out and was jotting something down in his slim notebook.

"Huh? Oh sure. But I hope you're still around to have any discussion. Well, if not, I guess I'll see you at the Resurrection."

Methodist Hospital was so strange to Virginia. She was used to the low brick suburban hospitals of home. Methodist was so much a part of the city, a totally urban environment. And their procedures were equally strange. Back home, if you were going in to the hospital, you would show up in the morning and they would be expecting you: your doctor would have made all the arrangements for you ahead of time. But here—she went to work on Wednesday morning and then waited for the hospital to call her to tell her when they had a bed ready. It was like standing in line for a movie, or waiting to rush through a revolving door.

Finally, in the mid-afternoon they called, and she and Fred took a taxi to Park Slope. They asked if she wanted a private or a semi-private room. At one time, when Fred was a successful commercial artist, they would have automatically opted for the private room. But now, with their minuscule monthly allowance, from the Witnesses, that was impossible. In fact, the Witnesses were paying for the entire operation, although they were under no obligation to do so: that was all the more reason to shun unnecessary luxury. But when she saw her "semi-private" accommodations she almost cried. For there were three other people in a large, sterile room. There was only a "shower curtain," as she called it, to provide privacy. Back home you would have to have been a pauper to get a room like this. At that moment she would have given anything to be back in Owensboro.

"Is there any way we can change this room?" Fred finally asked the nurse at the desk. He was distressed by Virginia's unhappiness.

The head nurse came back with the message: "There are no more private rooms available."

"But they told us at the desk . . ."

"That was half an hour ago," said the head nurse. "Good things disappear quickly around here."

Virginia got into her dressing gown and lay on the bed, trying not to listen to any of the three separate televisions going at the same time, or the wretched moans coming from out in the hallway.

A hospital administrator came by with a release form, a refusal to permit blood transfusions.

She dated it and signed it, and Fred signed it as well. The die was cast.

"Can I give you the sutures that I like?" asked Dr. Strong. "We'll start with 3–0 and 4–0 silk ties, 3–0 chromic, 4–0 nylon, and 2–0 silk for the Jackson-Pratt drains."

The pretty young O.R. nurse nodded. She had on false eyelashes and blue makeup, as if to concentrate all her cosmetics in the one small part of her body that was still visible.

"Listen, everybody. This is a Jehovah's Witness. Do you know what that means?" Strong asked.

"No blood," said a medical student.

"Precisely. No blood or blood products during or after the operation."

"What if she bleeds to death?" asked Berg, the resident who would be assisting Strong on the operation. "Couldn't we save her?"

"Well, that's highly unlikely," Strong said. "It's not really that dangerous an operation. But we couldn't even give her blood if we wanted to. Once she signed the release form, she was not typed and crossed." The resident nodded. All surgery patients are routinely "typed and crossed," that is, their blood is tested for its basic type and then cross-matched with specific bottles of donor blood to see if it reacts negatively with those particular specimens. In the case of Witnesses, however, the hospital would not permit such matching to be done, since it would indicate bad faith. No, Mrs. Gipe had burned her bridges behind her, as far as transfusions went. "What is possible," Strong added, "is undue blood loss, which could then cause complications in her recovery. But we're going to try to prevent that.

"Listen, we're going to go slow and easy," said Strong. "We'll try not to transect the pectoral. We'll open the clavical pectoral fascia. Identify the nerve first before you start cutting. Sometimes you get so carried away taking out these wonderful lymph nodes that before you know it you've severed something like an artery. That could be a bit . . . embarrassing in this case."

"Don't worry about me," said Berg. "I've done this plenty of times before."

They lifted Virginia's body from the wheeled stretcher onto the operating table. She helped scoot over, showing that the sedative hadn't completely taken effect. The anesthesiologist placed a big white patch containing an electronic sensor on her inner thigh and a nurse tucked her arms under the green sheets.

"I use a ten blade," Strong said to the resident. "Do you want to use a twenty?"

"No, I'll go with a ten."

"Did you give ethane?" he asked the anesthesiologist's resident.

"Yes."

"Pentathol? Oxygen?" He ran down the list of gases.

"It's highly overrated, that oxygen," said the resident, joking as usual.

As they adjusted the tube of gases and checked the readings on the Narkomy anesthesia system, there was some small talk about an O.R. party that Strong had missed. The nurses positioned the body and the lamp, draped Virginia, and began painting her with Povidone-iodine solution. Strong took part in the painting, making wide stripes of iodine on her breast, and actually pouring the solution on at one point straight from the stainless-steel mixing bowl. Then they marked the sections they were going to cut with Methylene blue solution.

After about half an hour of preparation, the two men—Strong and his resident—stood opposite each other, their green caps almost touching. One breast, the left, was exposed up to the shoulder and glistened under the theatrical lamp. Strong paused for a moment of silence—not to pray, but to steady his nerves and to reach deep inside himself for the inner strength that would carry him through three or four hours of intense, unrelieved tension. The scene around him was stark, almost Dali-esque, everything primary greens and blues and very, very white flesh.

Seven people stood around the body, but at this moment they worked as one organism, a team.

"Knife, please," he said suddenly. The nurse handed him a scalpel, and he made a cut straight across the breast, following the bluish-purple line the resident had painted on minutes earlier.

"We're doing a modified radical. I offered her a quadrant resection, but she turned it down. Too much risk of recurrence. I agree, but I didn't want to push her," said Strong.

"Retractor," said the resident, and he used the forklike instrument to pull back the flesh.

"Relax," said Strong to Berg. "What's your first name?"

"Arthur," said the resident.

"You're too strong for me in the morning, Arthur. I haven't had my breakfast yet."

The resident grasped several retractors now, pulling back

the flesh as Strong cut. They kept adding more retractors. "We'll give Dr. Hoffman something to work with," said Strong, referring to the reconstruction surgeon to whom he usually referred patients.

"Arthur, look. You can see where the tumor has infiltrated through the fascia. We want to take out these nodes and get them down to pathology for a frozen section. Also see if we can send a slip for estrogen receptors on what's left of this tumor." Estrogen receptors are markers on tumor cells that aid in prognosis and treatment planning.

A medical student stood off to one side. She seemed lost in thought.

Strong startled her back to reality with a question: "Why do we use sterile water to irrigate in operations such as this, rather than saline solution? Yes, you."

"I don't remember," she stammered.

"Answer: because it's hypotonic to cancer cells and causes them to burst."

The student decided to pay more attention to the operation. They had finished cutting down one purple line, revealing the breast tissue underneath. It was a peculiar yellow-orange, waxy substance, bumpy, with red blood oozing into the little valleys.

As they opened her up they had immediately clamped the small arteries involved, till at one point all flesh was obscured entirely by dangling metal clamps.

"Bovie," said Strong, asking for the electric knife. The current sizzled. He methodically applied the electrosurgical instrument to each clamp. It, in turn, conveyed the heat of the current to the small artery it held, sealing it off forever. They did this over and over again, methodically removing clamps as they went, until there was no more metal left.

The breast was now open and relatively dry for them to work on.

"We're going to have to go up and take out the tail as well," said Strong. The resident nodded. The "tail" was the portion of the breast that extended into the armpit of the woman. Most people were unaware it was even there, but in this case it could be critical, because the tumor had been practically sitting on the base of the tail itself.

"A long morning," the anesthesiologist's resident sighed.

"You in a hurry?" asked Strong. "Relax and watch what you're doing. I don't want any slipups."

"Look at these nodes," said Strong, sighing. "She's got a very high chance of having systemic disease. What does that mean?" he shot at the medical student.

"Systemic disease? It means the disease has spread beyond the original site, either through tissue infiltration, the blood system, or the lymph system—"

"Yes, but what does it mean for her prognosis and her treatment?"

"Well, the prognosis is poorer."

"Much poorer. And her treatment?"

"Chemotherapy?"

"Very good," said Strong, making an incision as he talked. "Usually a year of chemotherapy. Most commonly five-fluorouracil and methotrexate by injection, every week or two, and the patient takes Cytoxan by mouth. But it varies with the age and menstrual status of the patient. Sometimes they add prednisone to the mix. Different people do it different ways. She's also going to need a bone scan and a liver scan." These would show if the cancer had progressed already into those areas. If it had, the prognosis became even worse. There would be very little chance of curing the disease at this point—but the chemotherapy might help to retard it somewhat, Strong believed. It became an ethical issue at that point whether or not to recommend chemotherapy, since the possible prolongation of life would have to be weighed against the diminution in *quality* of life: the nausea, vomiting, hair loss, exhaustion.

Strong hoped this lady had some pull with the powers above to spare her from that fate.

They were working hard now—it was a long operation and you couldn't see the end of it when you first cut into the patient. This one would take longer because they had to be extra careful for bleeders.

"Number ten blade, please," Strong said, and the nurse handed it over. "Give me a little more juice on the Bovie. Coag on four, please. . . ." He burned a small vessel with the knife but was dissatisfied with the result. "Up it to five, please." The nurse adjusted the dials on the green electroknife console, a Valley Lab SSE2L.

Suddenly there was pandemonium. It was hard to say how it started.

Strong saw the jet of blood shoot up, felt its warmth on his hand, and one of the nurses cried out, more in surprise than fear, "Aaah! Aaah!"

Strong was yelling at the resident, "When you get to the fascia, don't cut! Just go down to the fascia! You have to go north. Slowly. One level at a time." The blood was spurting out of a severed artery.

The resident had regained his composure enough to try and soak it up with the surgical cloths. But it was coming out too fast and furious for Strong to even see it, much less get at it with the Bovie knife, which whined in his hand, eager for action.

"Clamp!" Strong yelled, and the metal tongs were in his hand almost before the word emerged.

"Arthur, get me a clear view of the vessel so I can clamp it." His face was white under the high-intensity lamp.

The resident daubed at the wound.

The bloody lap pads were being thrown one after another into the plastic-lined surgical bucket.

"We've got to get this," said Strong. He wrapped a cloth around his finger and probed deep into the wound.

Normally Strong would have called for a transfusion to be readied at this point. He rarely needed them, but it was a good feeling to have them as a backup. No matter how careful a surgeon was, he was not infallible and sometimes a vessel got cut. The thought of any harm coming to Mrs. Gipe naturally horrified him. But aside from the medical impossibility of giving blood at this point there was his word as a physician, his fiduciary bond, as they called it. He had given his word that he would not use blood. No, there was no alternative but to find the bleeder and seal it off.

"I think I've got it," said Strong, his face now red from the effort. Strong looked into the wound. He had poked a clamp in and by dint of sheer willpower and a great deal of luck—Mrs. Gipe might call it the presence of God—had gotten hold of the severed artery and clamped it off.

"Bovie," said Strong. "Coag."

The juice soared through the metal and burned away the dangling blood vessel in a puff of smoke.

They daubed around it until it was dry.

Strong let out his breath audibly and there was the laughter of relief in Operating Room #2.

"Good work," said Strong.

"I feel guilty," said Berg.

"Don't be ridiculous," said Strong, who liked the young doctor. "It happens. You're doing a fine job."

They resumed surgery, Strong cutting, and in a few more minutes there was nothing more said about it.

A few hours later the breast had been cleanly removed, two large flaps left for reconstruction. As Strong feared, the nodes had come back positive: she would need chemotherapy.

As they removed their bloody, sweaty clothing in the wash-up room, the medical student approached him.

"Doctor," she said, screwing up her courage, "may I ask you something?"

Strong smiled: they got younger and younger each year.

"Anything," he said, and he meant it. He was exhausted, but feeling good.

"Would you really have let her die back then? When she was bleeding, I mean."

He thought for a long moment. "I don't know. Rationally, I think I would have. That was our agreement. But emotionally . . . I just don't know. I'm a healer, not a killer. It's my job to cure people. It's really a dilemma, isn't it?" He paused, stripping off his transparent gloves and washing his hands. "To be honest with you, if it really came down to it, I think I would have had to let her go. She's a grown woman, and if that's her choice, I have to respect it."

The young girl shook her head slowly. "I think I'm going to go into pediatrics, or psychiatry. I can tell you one thing, Dr. Strong, anything but surgery!"

Virginia's recovery was rapid. Within a week she was able to return to her office in the new headquarters building overlooking the Brooklyn Bridge. She threw herself back into her tasks. Her job, by secular standards, was not a high position—unlike her husband, who had major responsibility for the production of the magazines. But to her it was important and consoling. And among the Witnesses in general there prevailed an egalitarianism modeled on the early Christian communities. For instance, when one Witness met another, they were discouraged from telling exactly what they did or comparing jobs. This was to prevent a top editor, say, from outranking a janitor or printer when it came to religious affairs. What did mundane rank matter when they were all bringing the good news of the Kingdom to the inhabited earth?

It was because of the pressing need of her religious tasks that Virginia tried to forget about the operation and threw herself back in the battle. Her arm felt stiff. With the modified radical such as she had received, there was no "bad" arm or "frozen shoulder," as sometimes happened with the old Halsted procedure. Nevertheless, the muscles were traumatized and retracted from the operation and needed exercises. Virginia felt some pain whenever she moved it vigorously, however, and so, instead of working the arm, she decided to leave it alone. Strong had warned her not to get an infection in that arm and not to allow blood to be drawn from it. This was to prevent swelling caused by the lack of draining lymph nodes in the armpit area. He also taught her deep-breathing exercises. She would lie on her back and breathe in very deeply, making her lower chest expand outward. Then she would relax and let the air out. She did this for about ten minutes. The purpose was to make the chest wall and the lungs expand, but it had an additional side effect: deep breathing was tremendously relaxing, and helped to clear her mind of the worries that were still troubling her. She wondered why she—indeed, why everyone—didn't practice these wonderful breathing exercises all the times, and not just at times like this. She remembered an old proverb she had heard: in heaven they teach you how to breathe. Wasn't that just like the illustrations in the *Watchtower*—and even more so the paintings from which they were derived and which were propped around the walls of the reception room on the fourth floor? Clean air, blue skies, with only small puffs of white clouds to highlight their perfection, the sun streaming down onto the peaceful families tending their gardens. What a contrast to the smog and pollution of a city like New York! It was more like she remembered her childhood in Owensboro to have been—a clean time, a simple time. Truly, when God's Kingdom was restored, the earth would again be clean and simple and everyone could then breathe the way they were intended to.

Dr. Strong had said that a volunteer from a recovered-patients' organization would visit her in the hospital, but they never came, and she was too busy to find out why. She did the best she could in the office. She tried moving her arm upward, toward her head, but it hurt and she pulled back. She was afraid of pushing too far, of tearing the stitches.

Her armpit and chest felt stiff and tight. She tried lifting a mug in the office, but found that difficult. Finally, she was able to get her arm out at eye level. She also practiced regaining those simple motions that are taken so much for granted: washing and brushing her hair, fastening her bra, reaching into cabinets and closets. Often she had to get Fred to help her remove something from a shelf she could not reach. But she felt she was making definite progress and was sure Dr. Strong would be pleased. The wound was healing nicely and she was back into her normal routine. She was, in short, the admiration of all her colleagues.

When she visited Dr. Strong on the following Thursday evening, he was indeed pleased with her healing. Strong had no doubt that she would spring back quickly from the operation. He explained to her the purpose and program of the Breast Health Program and asked her to join.

"Well, as a Witness, Dr. Strong, I'm not really supposed to join any outside organizations. We recognize only one organization, and that is the Church of Jehovah. We don't recognize any government known to Man."

Strong nodded: he remembered that in high school there had been two kids, both Jehovah's Witnesses, who had refused to salute the flag or pledge allegiance. In the paranoid fifties, that was almost equivalent to being a Communist, and they had been given a hard time. Once again he marveled at the dedication of these people, who almost seemed to court persecution for the sake of their faith.

"On the other hand," she said, sensing his obvious disappointment, "I certainly subscribe to the goals of the Breast Health Program. I'll come and see you on the schedule you suggest, read the *Bulletin,* and, don't worry, I'll send other people to you if they need care."

Strong nodded and thanked her: he felt a special responsibility to these Witnesses. For many doctors, they were medical outcasts because of their stand on blood, and the danger of them neglecting their breast problems seemed to him very pressing.

"Okay, now let's see how well you've recovered use of that arm," he said. "Complete shoulder motion is achieved when you are able to reach across your head and touch your opposite ear without feeling any pain or stretching sensations in your armpit." Virginia reached up, but it was immediately painful. In her own exercise she had never gone so far—she had been afraid to. She made a heroic effort and tried to reach her ear by going around the back of her head.

"No! No! No!" Strong yelled. "That's cheating. Don't try to sneak your arm behind your head. Keep your head up and bring your upper arm parallel to your ear. Then reach over." Strong knew what the problem was: She was simply afraid to move her arm.

Virginia tried again, but she knew even before starting that she would fail.

"What's wrong with you?" Strong asked. "Why haven't you been doing your exercises?"

"But I have been," Virginia said, almost on the point of tears. She was abashed at her failure and felt humiliated by his attitude.

"Okay, try this then," said Strong. "Raise your arms as high as you can over your head. Keep the upper part of your arms touching your ears as you do it."

Virginia took a deep breath and then reached upward. Her elbows remained crooked and her hands barely went over her head at all.

Strong was very concerned. Although Mrs. Gipe said she subscribed to the goals of the BHP, she was clearly also lacking in confidence. "I imagine that people have told you that you lose the use of your shoulder after a mastectomy. But this is just no longer true with the kind of procedure you had. Try to relax a little bit. I want you to do these exercises so that the scar doesn't stiffen up on you, that's all."

"But I do exercise regularly," she said in frustration. "Every day. Three times a day, in fact. But I don't want to snap or tear anything. I mean, after all, I'm doing this all on my own, I haven't had any help, and so I've just done the best I could under the circumstances."

"What do you mean, 'all on your own?' " Strong asked suspiciously. "What about the volunteers? Why haven't you followed their recommendations?"

"What volunteers?" said Virginia, in a tone of voice that—for her, at least—constituted a veritable shout.

Strong suddenly realized what had happened. "You mean you didn't get to talk to a volunteer from the recovered patients?"

Virginia shook her head.

"Jesus Christ," Strong hissed, but then he blushed, realizing he had used the expletive in the wrong company. Virginia smiled. She had heard it before.

"I mean, I'm sorry. How could I be so stupid? I'm really sorry. It's just that I thought . . ."

"No, I never saw them," said Virginia, trying not to enjoy her vindication too much.

"They're usually very good. Maybe it was my fault," said Strong. "They would tell you all about how to do this. Why don't you come to the Breast Health Program, then? We can provide you with the same information."

"In that case," said Virginia. "Tomorrow morning I will be at the office at nine o'clock. And I won't come back here, Dr. Strong, until my arm's back to normal. I promise you that."

At the Breast Health Program office, the nurses gave her a kit of information and some paraphernalia including a soft rubber ball and a six-foot length of rope. She actually came to enjoy some of the exercises. When she was getting up and at night before retiring, she lay flat holding the rubber ball in her hand. She then lifted her arm straight up, as the nurse in the BHP office had shown her, and alternately squeezed and relaxed it. Sometimes it was uncomfortable for her to hold the arm straight up and so she used several pillows to support the arm as she performed the task. This was supposed to be useful in preventing swelling in the affected limb.

She took the six-foot length of rope home with her. She had

gotten permission of the building superintendant to have a handyman drive a large nail into the top edge of her closet door, about six inches from the outside corner. The hotel-type rooms were so neat and pristine that she hated the thought of damaging them in any way; it upset her that now the closet door couldn't close, but the janitor assured her that the hole at the top would never been seen. In a short while, after she had achieved mastery of her condition, the nail could be removed.

Virginia tied knots on each end of the rope and threw it over the top of the door with her "good" arm, looping it around the nail. She then sat with her legs hugging the two sides of the door firmly and kept the soles of her feet planted firmly on the floor. She held the ends of the rope in each hand and, as instructed, she put the knots between her third and fourth fingers.

Very slowly she raised the affected arm as far as she could by pulling down on the rope with her other arm. She kept the raised arm as close to her head as she could manage. She then reversed the motion and raised the "good" arm by pulling with the affected one. She rested, and then repeated this exercise for about fifteen minutes, or as long as she could stand it.

The purpose of this pulley exercise was to increase the forward motion of her shoulder, which was still a bit stiff from the scar of the operation.

Virginia also did other exercises. In her office she was able to do "hand wall-climbing." She would stand facing the wall, six to nine inches from the baseboard. She would then bend her elbows and place her palms against the wall at shoulder level. She would work both her hands up the wall in a climbing motion, marking the spot with a bit of tape so that she could check her progress. Each day she attempted to go a few inches higher.

This was exhausting after a while, so she would relax by resting her head against the wall. The purpose of this, they said, was to increase the forward motion of her shoulders.

She also did the back-scratcher exercise, to be able to reach into the middle of her back, and the elbow pull-in, to increase the rotation of her shoulder in both directions.

Two weeks later she went to see Dr. Strong. He examined her scar and then nervously asked to see if she could touch the top of her head. Virginia reached around nimbly and touched her head and then continued on and touched her other ear.

Then, without his asking, she reached her arms upward above her head. The exercises had paid off. She could perform this and any other task Strong asked her to do with only a small amount of pulling sensation in the shoulder.

"This is incredible," said Strong, shaking his head. "What are you doing, getting ready for the Olympics?"

"I just didn't want you to be disappointed in me, Doctor," she said, smiling. "Or for me to be disappointed in myself."

Robin

Of all the aspects of cancer treatment, the one that frightened Robin the most was chemotherapy. Surgery she could deal with—once finished, it was over and done with. Even radiation wasn't so bad. But chemotherapy frightened her. There was something about the idea of the injection of poisons into her veins that unnerved her, no matter how good the therapeutic purpose. People threw the odds, the figures, the statistics at her. But somehow this part of it seemed the most unreal of all.

She was sitting in the office of Dr. Vogel, an oncologist on Park Avenue. "Oncologist" was a new word in her vocabulary. She had looked it up in the big dictionary she had gotten as a present in high school, but it wasn't there. From what she could see, an "oncologist" was a fancy word for chemotherapist. It sounded better, she thought. Anything sounds better than chemotherapist.

The office itself surprised her. The first thing she noticed was how big it was. It looked like a waiting room of a small hospital. She was impressed. There were padded plastic seats and neatly arranged couches—everything in soothing greens and yellows. Chagall posters, all in the same frames. She thought she had seen the same posters on sale, fully framed in chrome, in a discount print shop on Third Avenue. How depressing!

The secretaries sat answering phones behind an oval-shaped desk. They had faces ready to smile—a mere glance triggered off a grin, a sympathetic happy face.

A bald man emerged, white coat trailing, and grabbed the phone.

"Did you get the toxoplasmosis titre . . . ?" he asked. "It's negative. Same symptoms?" A pause. "I didn't see anything biopsable." That was another new word. Robin cringed into the corner of her couch.

A woman stood writing a check by the desk. ("Fees Are Due and Payable Upon Completion of Visit.") She pleaded with the doctor, who was trying to finish his call.

"Please, can't I wait another week? I don't want to come the day after the holiday."

"It's really not—" the doctor began.

"Please—"

"Look," he said impatiently. "I can't tell you what to do or not do, but optimally you should come in."

Levolor blinds. The hushed sound of the air handlers, neither too hot nor too cold. The nurse putting cold cream on her hands. Beyond the desk she could see a kind of picture window and beyond that, row after row of glass bottles filled with chemicals. That was the bottom line, she thought, and all this good cheer was just illusionary trappings.

But she stayed. And in reality, the main reason she stayed was because of her growing attachment to Leslie Strong. She didn't want to disappoint him. The least she could do was talk to this Dr. Vogel.

When they called her name she was ushered into a small white examining room. God, how she hated these damn doctors' offices and sterile examining rooms. Dr. Vogel came in and sat himself opposite her. He was the same man she had seen ten minutes before on the phone.

"So, you're a patient of Dr. Strong's," he began. "You're in the Breast Health Program. Good. I've gone over your case very carefully with Dr. Strong. In our opinion, as he's explained to you, you're a candidate for adjuvant chemotherapy."

"Take it one step back," said Robin, asserting herself. "I'm here to assess the possibility of undertaking chemotherapy." She knew big words, too! "But you'll have to take it from square one and explain everything to me, or I'll—" She was about to say something like "take my business elsewhere," but she realized what she was saying was coming out hostile. "—or I just won't understand it."

"Fine," said Vogel. "Well, then, there are two types of cancer chemotherapy, basically. There is chemotherapy given for existing disease and chemotherapy given as a protection *against* the disease coming back. Now, in your case, Robin—may I call you Robin?" She nodded. "In your case, the tumor was removed and so were the lymph nodes. As you know, many of them came up positive, but by all the other tests—bone scan, liver scan, and so forth, there is no evidence of any disease.

"So you might think that you are free and clear. But the problem is that statistically we know that a high percentage of patients with tumor in the regional lymph nodes—the armpits—will eventually develop cancer in distant sites as well. As a matter of fact, Robin, I have some patients with uninvolved lymph nodes who are also receiving chemotherapy because of certain other signs that indicate a relapse is likely. Are you following so far?"

His manner was didactic, a bit condescending, perhaps, but she was interested and nodded: after all, it was her life he was talking about. She might as well listen.

"So why is that?" he asked rhetorically. "It's obvious—both logically and from studies that have been carried out—that the disease must already be present in other areas of the body at the time of the mastectomy, despite negative blood chemistry tests, negative X rays and negative scans of various organs."

"Are you saying I still have cancer?"

"Well, you don't have *clinical* cancer, that we know. But you may have small colonies of cells—small in this case can be anywhere up to millions of cells, you understand—which are growing at a geometrical rate. There's no way to find these with today's technology, much less operate on them. And so, in order to reduce the chance of the disease recurring, we treat patients with adjuvant or protective chemotherapy. Are you still following this?"

"I guess so," said Robin. "I know a little bit about the topic," said Robin. "My mother had breast cancer; she died of it. I saw the chemo patients—the sores all over their mouths, whew! That was really bad. The hair falling out . . ."

Vogel waved his hand. "That's why I started out by telling you the distinction between chemotherapy as a treatment for existing disease and chemotherapy as a preventive. I agree, the treatment for existing disease can be very trying—"

"To put it mildly," she interjected.

"—because the doses are so high. But those patients are dying of their disease and these are what we call heroic measures. But as a preventive we generally use much smaller doses of the Cooper regimen, also called CMF-VP: this is a combination of Cytoxan, methotrexate, five-fluorouracil, vincristine, and prednisone."

"How often do—would I have to take this?"

"Well, the first eight days of each month, with Cytoxan given by mouth the first fourteen days of each month. This office treatment is continued for a number of monthly cycles, depending on the particular case."

"What're the side effects?" Robin asked nervously.

"This regimen has minimum nausea and vomiting—"

"Great," said Robin, shaking her head.

Vogel smiled. He had a warm smile, Robin thought. He should use it more often.

"Well, it's minimal," said Vogel. "Most of my patients, Robin, are able to continue to work on the job or around the house. The other side effects, like hair loss, are uncommon and are completely reversible."

"At least you're being frank with me. But, tell me, if I do undertake this regimen, do you think my chances will really be improved? I mean, am I free and clear if I go through a course of this stuff?"

Vogel laughed. "I wish I could promise you that," he said. "But the chance of recurrence is related to various factors such as the number of lymph nodes involved; the extent of nodal involvement, that is, how much of the lymph node is replaced by tumor; the position of the positive lymph nodes; the size of the primary tumor; and the menopausal status."

He thought for a minute: most of Robin's prognostic factors were negative. She had a large tumor with many nodes involved. The one bright spot was her menopausal status. "In your case, it's greatly in your favor that you are pre-menopausal. We have a better success rate in women like you."

"So Leslie told me," she said. "It seems everybody's reading from the same script these days. But what you haven't told me is what happens if I take the treatments, and then a month or a year or ten years later the cancer *still* comes back. What the hell do I do then?"

Vogel looked away for a moment. He hated this question, but it always came up.

"Well, unfortunately, that happens sometimes," he said in a low voice. He had seen enough of them. In fact, he generally got to see them all, since the oncologist is usually sent exactly those cases the surgeon can no longer help. That was why, for Vogel, adjuvant cases, like Robin's, were the most encouraging part of his practice.

"The first thing we do is evaluate these patients to see if the tumor can be influenced by hormone alternation. You probably don't know this, but at the time of your surgery, Dr. Strong had your tissues analyzed for what is called estrogen and progesterone receptors. In your case these were positive, and so that gives us another weapon in the fight against the disease—a weapon we're going to keep in reserve and hope we don't have to use."

"So you mean you'd give me some kind of anti-hormone to knock out my female hormones?"

"Well, it's not quite that simple," said Vogel. "I mean, in women there is a whole sequence of hormonal treatments depending mainly on the relationship to menopause. In the premenopausal patient, like yourself, this may involve direct surgical removal of the ovaries or radiation to the glands. This sometimes results in a halt of the growth of the tumors. You have probably heard that, in the forties, they thought this was a magical treatment for cancer. But the problem is that the cancer eventually returns. When it does, the progressive growth of the tumor can again be halted or reversed by administering a male hormone, or by a drug that suppresses the adrenal gland."

"And if these all fail?" asked Robin nervously.

"Well, if hormone-manipulative therapy such as tomoxifin fails, we still have some other drugs that can affect the tumor. But you have to understand, Robin, we're not here to perform miracles. We're doing the best we can do with what we have. Nor should you let this kind of talk scare you, because your chances of controlling the disease with a very minimal kind of chemotherapy are, in my opinion, very good.

"You're also lucky that you're in the BHP. You'll have Strong checking up on you every month or so, and I'm in touch with him every day or two. If any problems develop, you can count on us to coordinate our treatment and do the best we can do for you."

Two weeks after her surgery, Robin began chemotherapy. She went to Vogel's office in the afternoon and he gave her a big injection of drugs—methotrexate and 5-fluorouracil. She also took his pills—Cytoxan. And, surprise of surprises, little happened, at least at first.

She felt a bit nauseous the days of the injection, but nothing she couldn't live with. Her beautiful amber hair started to thin, but not so much that she had to wear one of those tell-tale kerchiefs around her head. Life went on. She continued to walk Barnie, her pooch, the honorary mayor of East 83rd Street. She continued to water her plants, which, after ten years of growth, covered one whole wall of her sunlit tenth-floor apartment. She continued to play the piano and the drums, to the chagrin of her neighbors. Although she knew everyone in the building and, after ten years, practically everyone on the block, few knew about her operation. Those who had heard were funny. She'd catch them sneaking glances at her bosom, trying to figure out which one was gone.

Peter gave her what she called his "locker-room speech."

"We've been together in the good times, babe, and now that some bad times've come, we'll weather the storm and stick together through them as well."

It was corny, but she ate it up.

Sex was only strange because so little had changed between them. At first she walked around with a robe on, but he objected strenuously. With good instincts he knew that she had to accept the fact of the mastectomy in order to forget about it. And so she slowly disrobed for him the first time.

After a long pause, he said, with mock seriousness, "Well, it's not like you've given up that much. Big tits were never your strong suit." She loved him for it, and would have cringed at some dreadful platitude.

And in some ways she felt lucky. She was hardly scarred at all. Leslie Strong had done a magnificent job on her. Her mother, on the other hand, had been scarred—terribly. They had really botched her up. That was what she dreaded, and so the long, straight line down her chest was something of a relief and almost—in a funny way—a matter of pride. "I'm a walking work of art," she once told Strong, who couldn't quite get used to her unconventional sense of humor or way of life.

In bed with Peter, things were the same as ever. Everything still "worked." On the surface, at least, it was like nothing had happened.

Underneath, there were changes taking place, changes she didn't quite understand or yet know how to deal with.

On Robin's wall was a plaque that a friend of hers had given her years before. It was engraved on a piece of wood—a poem he had written that had summed up her view of her very "sixties-type" lifestyle. It read:

> *A falling pebble*
>   *can start an avalanche*
> *An unseen root*
>   *can destroy a forest*
> *Nothing is safe from pain*
> *Nothing lasts forever*
> *In view of such*
>   *impermanence*
> *What choice but to live*
>   *from day to day*
> *Stealing from life*
>   *all one can carry.*

It still seemed true to her—truer, in fact, than when she first fell in love with it—especially the part about the "falling pebble" and the "unseen root." The unseen root had certainly been growing underneath her.

But on the other hand, she wasn't sure she could go on living from day to day anymore, as she had done for over ten years. She felt a deep pull—not exactly toward bourgeois respectability, but toward some kind of stability and achievement. She wanted to do something with her life, *make* something. She also wanted to have children. At thirty-three, she was getting perilously close to the point of no return. But she knew she would have to wait until she was free and clear of these chemo drugs before she could do that. Her life had changed. Although she was still Peter Pan, and still did not really believe she would ever grow up (much less die), some new note had crept into her life. It was a bass note, to be sure, yet surprisingly it was not an entirely unpleasant change.

Later that summer, when her roommate was on vacation, Peter came to stay with her for several weeks. Lately there had indeed been some changes, but not the kind she had intended. "Wonder Woman," who had withstood the chemotherapy without a flinch, was slowly weakening. It was not something she could pinpoint. Peter pressed her for an explanation. He was a draughtsman and liked precision in instruments and people.

"I can't explain it," Robin said, wrinkling her forehead. "It's not exactly the nausea, not exactly the hair loss. Not exactly my loss of control over my bodily functions, although that's disturbing. I just feel so *weak* and *shitty* all the time. Like I'm being poisoned."

"Well, you are," said Peter, with typical exactitude. "Chemotherapy is a poison, deliberately designed to poison the cancer cells and leave as many normal cells as possible unaffected."

His almost cheerful acceptance of this scientific wonder bothered her. She hated to disagree with him, but her nature was so different from his that they often quarreled.

"Sounds great, Peter, the way you say it."

"I'm sure it's unpleasant," said Peter. "However, if it works to kill the cancer cells, then I'm glad you're doing it."

She wondered if he would be quite so sanguine if it was him going in there week after week to get that tube in his arm.

"Come on," she said after a few minutes of this, "let's stop quarreling. It's a beautiful day out. Let's go for a walk."

Robin picked up a dozen eggs from a small place she had discovered, one of the few fresh poultry places left on the island of Manhattan. "You haven't had eggs until you've tasted these," she said, with some of her old enthusiasm.

They crossed East End Avenue, where Leslie Strong lived,

and went down to the park along the river. The river looked gorgeous—urban and urbane. Even the utilitarian Triboro Bridge looked romantic. Seagulls swirled overhead; the currents of Hell's Gate made Van Gogh–esque curlicues in the water. The park was almost deserted on a Friday afternoon. Robin said hello to the manager of the local supermarket's vegetable department, out for a late lunchtime stroll. Her dog exchanged intimate sniffs with a few other pooches off their leashes.

They were deep in a conversation about something that had happened to them at Fire Island when Robin realized she had to go to the bathroom. She looked around for a comfort station, but there was none. She could see that the gate of the reconstructed Fire Boat House was locked.

"I have to find a restroom," she said suddenly.

"Oh, okay. But do you remember how you . . ."

"Peter, I'm serious! You don't understand. I've got to get to the bathroom quick."

"Oh, all right," said Peter, somewhat annoyed. He couldn't understand what the great urgency was. "We'll head back."

They started to walk up the path, passing an old man feeding the brown squirrels. Barney trotted along behind them, seemingly more alarmed than her boyfriend by the sudden change of pace.

"I don't believe this," said Robin, suddenly alarmed. "I don't believe what these damn drugs are doing to me."

And it had to happen in front of Peter, of all people. If it had been her roommate, she could have handled it, but not Peter. It was impossible to explain, but she hated to have him see her like this.

Robin looked around desperately for a bathroom. She remembered one time when she had been a kid on a day-camp trip. The movement of the bus, the fumes, had gotten to her and she had to go, but the bus driver would not stop. When they finally made it to the state park, she had made in her pants, and the other kids had hooted her all the way to the smelly toilets.

There was a brick sanitation house in the distance. They hurried to it, Robin's face covered with sweat, but when they got there, it, too, was locked. Off in the distance were the apartment houses of East End Avenue, including, ironically, Leslie Strong's at the end of the row. Perhaps she could go there, although she knew he wouldn't be home in the midafternoon. Perhaps there would be a store, a restaurant. . . .

"Pete," she said, "what should I do? I can't hold it in."

"Go in the bushes," said Peter. "I'll keep lookout."

"There're people all around," she whispered.

Suddenly the struggle was over. Her light-gray running pants turned a dull leaden color and the urine ran down her leg into her tennis shoes. She started sobbing hysterically, uncontrollably.

"Christ, Robin," said Peter. "What's the big deal? It's a natural thing. It's not your fault."

She still sobbed, but less so.

"You can't help it. You're under the influence of drugs and it's screwed up your system. But soon you'll be off them and you'll get back to normal."

He sounded like he meant it, too. In fact, she couldn't quite believe her ears. Was this really her boyfriend speaking? She had never seen him quite so understanding before. But time changed people, and not always for the worse.

"You're sweet," she blubbered. "I love you."

"Cut that out," he said half-jokingly. "Don't start getting sentimental on me."

She laughed. It *was* the same old Peter. But she loved him even more, for his real concern for her had shown through his often cold exterior.

"Just stay here, Rob. I'll run back to the apartment and get you a blanket or something. A new pair of pants."

"Oh, the hell with it," she said. "We'll just jog back to the apartment. It's only a few blocks now. If anyone asks I'll just say I got caught under the lawn sprinklers."

The three of them—Robin, Peter, and Barney—trotted out of the park and through the traffic of First Avenue. Robin was soaked from the waist down. The rest of New York went about its business and, as usual, nobody noticed a thing.

PART FOUR
Autumn

Gladys

The lump in Gladys' left breast would not go away. Now when she showered she could not help reaching up and touching herself there. Was she imagining it, or was it growing more prominent?

Finally Polly convinced her to call the American Cancer Society and ask for the name of a doctor who would do a two-phase operation. They gave her the number of Dr. Leslie Strong. Strong's answering service picked up the call because he was operating.

"Give me an appointment for the evening," she told them. "I don't want to have to interrupt work."

They gave her an evening appointment for the next day and his address on East End Avenue. When she arrived at the address with her husband, however, she found herself face to face with a teenage boy. It was Strong's home address she had gotten. His son David, perplexed, had answered the door. He called his father's office and half an hour later Gladys was sitting in Strong's office on 72nd Street.

Strong was abashed when he heard about his answering service's mistake. Such foul-ups alarmed him. On the one hand, as a surgeon he *had* to be orderly—there were just no two ways about it. You couldn't go leaving sponges or clips in patients, or missing appointments and the like. On the other hand, with his two practices—in Brooklyn and Manhattan—and his time-consuming work on the Breast Health Program—soliciting business subscribers, enlisting doctors, writing the newsletter, appearing on television and radio—and, of course, seeing patients—he was running himself ragged. What is more, his two children, who lived during the week with their mother in Queens, were entering adolescence, and were presenting him with more time-consuming needs and challenges all the time. Then for something like this to happen . . . he would have to have a stern talk with the answering service, and find a new one, if need be.

Gladys repeated the story of what had happened to her at the cancer center and Strong secretly found it amusing. She also said something else of no importance to her, but of great significance to him. She mentioned casually that she was a family friend of Dr. McCardle. It was precisely because of the closeness of this relationship that she did not want him to operate on her. Yet McCardle was one of the "gods" of breast surgery in New York. She couldn't have devised a better calling card for herself if she had tried.

When Strong examined her and took her history, however, he became a bit alarmed. The tumor was hard and, although small, seemed firmly rooted in its spot. What is more, he learned that Gladys' mother had died of cancer at thirty-eight. That was many years before, and no one seemed to know what kind of cancer it was.

Mrs. Kalin's attitude also disturbed him. She was certainly "a tough old dame," as she referred to herself. But she also was very vulnerable, sensitive, and—the key word—scared. She had an almost morbid fear of surgery, which so far had kept her from getting adequate advice. In his eyes, the earlier surgeon's behavior was reprehensible, but quite in keeping with the old-fashioned professional's attitude about not allowing the patient to choose her own therapy. Of course, the reasons for doing this were obvious to him: a two-stage operation meant an extra expenditure of time, money, and hospital resources. In addition, to allow the patient to decide on the course of treatment alternatives after a biopsy left open the possibility that she would choose to go elsewhere. But the advantages to Strong greatly outweighed the drawbacks: it largely came down to a philosophical difference. Whose body was it, and whose right to make the ultimate decision? To Strong, that right would always lie with the patient, and he hoped that he would never grow so powerful or all-mighty that he thought otherwise.

He wanted to be sympathetic and understanding to Gladys, but she also frightened him, since she was obviously quite capable of walking away from the problem for another couple of months or even years, until it would be too late.

"Let's play it by ear," he said tentatively. "The first thing is to have a biopsy."

"A biopsy," she said uncertainly. "How about a needle, Dr. Strong? Why can't you do it with a needle, or with injections? You understand, I don't want to be operated on. In fact, I'm gonna do anything I have to not to be cut open."

Strong stood his ground and argued back, urging the danger of delay.

"I respect what you're saying, but I don't intend to be operated on," Gladys countered. "I hate hospitals. I hate to stay in them. If you're sick, I'll come visit you, but otherwise, uh uh."

"Look," said Strong, getting stern. "If you want somebody to just agree with you I can get you some idiot around the corner. If you come to me, you're coming for my professional advice, and I'm telling you, there's no way you're going to get out of this without an operation."

The two of them faced each other as if over a negotiating table. Neither of them was going to give way easily. Finally Gladys said, "Well, maybe just a biopsy. At least you talk to me and don't walk away the way the other slob did. But I'm warning you. I'm not staying overnight in the hospital. Not at all. I'll come in, you'll do your thing, and I'll be out of there like a shot."

Strong shrugged his shoulders. Outpatient breast biopsies were not that unusual, but because of the position and depth of the tumor he did not advise it in this case. And because it was a bit unconventional, if she developed an infection or complications later, then everyone, from the hospital administrator to the family, would be down on him. Worst of all, McCardle would certainly hear about it, and word would get around about Strong's walkaway patient. But what was the other alternative? To let her go back to New Jersey and die of an uncontrolled spreading carcinoma (assuming it was carcinoma, which was his intuition)?

It was a dilemma quite typical of this profession, the choice between two unattractive alternatives.

"Okay," he said, "you win." He hoped she would see it that way. "You're a hell of a fighter. You can leave the same day. Just be sure you're at the hospital at seven-thirty in the morning. I'll do you around noon, and you can go home in the afternoon if you feel well enough."

When she left the office and was heading home on the Interstate 80 Expressway, she said to Sam, "I can't believe I let that bastard talk me into it! He's got an honest face, but he's one hell of a clever talker, if you ask me. I just hope they don't sneak me the 'black bottle' while I'm in there."

"You're gonna be all right, Gladys," said Sam. "But only if you listen to the doctor. You don't know anything about medicine, let's face it. Just let them tell you what to do and then do it."

For Sam it was all a bit bewildering. They had only been married a short time. He had known Gladys in the Bronx, when his wife and her husband were still alive. There had never been anything between them at that time, of course. They were just friends.

Gladys wasn't the easiest person in the world to live with, but he enjoyed their life together in her big house in Jersey. And now this.

"Don't worry about me, Sam," Gladys said. "I'm not going to let them push me around. Gladys knows how to take care of herself!"

"I know," said Sam humorously. "That's just what I'm worried about."

Gladys woke up quickly after the biopsy. She lay in the recovery room of Beth Israel, staring at the ceiling. Squinting her eyes, she could see that it was almost 2:00 P.M. The operation had taken no more than an hour, and so she must have been asleep for another hour here.

She lay motionless, in that peculiar twilight state, for a long moment, until she was startled by the ripping sound of the curtain being drawn back. It was Dr. Strong.

"Gladys, I want to talk to you," he began.

"You don't have to bother, Dr. Strong," she said, her voice mingling tears and tenderness. "You're a very bad cardplayer. I can see it in your face." His face, with its deep worry lines, was, in fact, quite transparent: he was groping for words, trying to figure out how to break it to her. And so she solved the problem by breaking it to him:

"It's malignant, isn't it?" she said.

He nodded. "It is. We're going to have to remove it." "It" meant, of course, the breast.

Some people cry in this situation, or moan, or even thrash about. Gladys simply said, quickly, "I don't want to think about this. Okay," she added in a businesslike tone, "I want to go home now."

Strong was reluctant to have her leave, but that was the bargain he had struck in order to get her into the hospital in the first place, and he intended to abide by it.

"Fine," he said, "but you'll have to stay for an hour to let the effects of the anesthetic wear off."

"I don't need to wait," said Gladys.

Strong looked around for help, but found none. "Your husband's not here," he said finally.

"I don't need anybody," she shot back, propping herself up on her elbow. "I'll call a cab to the train station and then grab a taxi right at the station and I'll be home."

The recovery room nurse smiled, but walked away. Strong continued to reason with Gladys, but with little success. No matter what he said, she came right back to her theme: I want to go home! Finally her husband, Sam, came to the door of the recovery room and peeked in. Since the sign said no visitors were allowed, he rapped lightly on the window.

Strong tried to reason with him, too, but Sam just shrugged his shoulders, meaning "You don't argue with Gladys Kalin."

"You have to lie down," said Strong, as Gladys tried to right herself and swing her legs over the side of the bed.

"I'm perfectly awake, doctor," she shot back. "Listen, I'm so upset about this thing that I want to go home."

Strong's air call went off with a startling beep.

"I've got to go," he said. "I have another operation. But I want you to stay put for just an hour."

When he left, Gladys immediately said to the nurse, "Help me up onto the floor."

"You'll fall down," said the nurse, no longer smiling, since the problem had now been dumped in her lap.

"I can walk," Gladys shouted.

"You cannot," the nurse shouted back.

Gladys finally settled the argument by jumping out of the bed, with an agility that surprised and alarmed the nurse. She grabbed the I.V. drip and its stand in one hand and started walking, or at least wobbling, around the recovery room.

"Jeez, I look like Father Time," she quipped. Suddenly she said, "Listen, nurse, I feel a little nauseous. I haven't eaten since nine o'clock last night. What time is it? Almost three P.M. already. No wonder I'm nauseous. Be a dear and make me a cup of something."

She sat down on the edge of the bed. There was a pot of yellowish hot water in the nurses' lounge that adjoined the recovery room. The nurse made her a cup of tea, light, and brought it to her.

"Mmm, this feels good, this tastes good," said Gladys. She drank it down. About fifteen seconds later she suddenly got a peculiar look on her face and vomited it up onto the floor, her retching blending with the moans and groans of the other semiconscious patients.

The nurse ran and got some towels to mop it up. "Now you've got to stay," she said with new authority.

"That's what you think," said Gladys, who was still panting from the effort. "I just threw up because I hadn't eaten. Also the anesthetics. But I'm better now. Listen, it's a lot more aggravating sitting here than being home. What am I going to do here? Listen to the other patients in their misery?" It was true, in a sense: the noises from the other patients were depressing. The nurse hardly heard them anymore because she was surrounded by them for at least eight hours a day.

"Listen, at least let me get dressed. Let me get started, and that'll take about thirty minutes. Strong left almost half an hour ago, and so that makes an hour."

"Dr. Strong meant one hour from the time you felt better."

"I know I'm being a pain in the whatever. But be a doll and

go get me my clothing. I swear I'm well. My husband's right outside the door. He'll help me."

"Why don't you just stay overnight," said the nurse, "like everybody else?"

" 'Cause I'm not like everybody else. Hospitals make me nervous. They give me anxiety. Look at it this way: you'll get rid of me, and I'll be one less to worry about."

The nurse laughed. *That* argument was irresistible!

And, in the end, Gladys won: She got her clothing and was walking out of the door at First Avenue and 16th Street, by 4:00 P.M.

Going out, Gladys ran into a lady she had met whose son had gone in for a polyps operation. The woman had rattled on and on about anything and everything. Anxiety makes people talk, Gladys had thought. It'll do her good to get it off her chest.

Now the lady was smiling. "Not cancer, not cancer," she said to Gladys, making a V-for-victory sign. She neglected to ask how Gladys had made out, probably figuring that if she was walking out self-confidently her operation must have turned out equally well.

And that was all right with Gladys. She didn't need anybody's pity.

Strong offered Gladys a choice of two operative procedures. She could have a modified radical mastectomy, or a quadrantectomy. After seeking a second opinion and talking to McCardle on the phone, she opted for the mastectomy. This was a phenomenon Strong had seen quite often. Even when more conservative procedures, such as the quadrantectomy, were available as options, many women still went for the "tried and true" mastectomy. The same had been true when the modified radical (which spared the chest-wall muscle) had begun to replace the more drastic Halsted procedure. Many women stuck with the Halsted, even though it left them without an important muscle. Yet the new, more sparing procedures had been shown to be as safe and effective as the Halsted operation.

Gladys's mastectomy went off without incident. Strong removed twenty-five of her lymph nodes (the number of lymph nodes varied from person to person) and only one of them turned out to be malignant. But the tumor itself had been over two centimeters in diameter. Given these factors, it was Strong's opinion that chemotherapy would be advisable in Gladys's case. He would arrange for her to see Dr. Vogel the following week, but he knew that she might give him trouble over it. One good sign was that her estrogen and progesterone receptors were positive—always a hopeful prognostic sign.

Gladys awoke from the operation in a crush of pain. It felt like an elephant had been parading up and down her chest. She couldn't describe it to Sam, who sat at her bedside, a *Daily News* in his lap, unsure of what to do. Her mouth was parched and she complained of aches everywhere—in her bones, in her arms and legs, in her lungs. She wasn't talking now about leaving the hospital. She just rolled over and went back to sleep, weeping silently.

The next day, however, the pain wasn't all that bad—at least it was bearable, and focused now in her chest. She pulled back the covers and glanced briefly at herself. The bandages were so bulky that for a moment her heart leaped. Maybe it had all been a mistake, and they had left her with her breast after all! Somehow, going into the operation, she had believed that it was all a bad dream. This wasn't really happening. It *couldn't* be happening, not to her. She would come to, and everyone would be laughing—we made a mistake. But then she touched the bandage and felt the hollowness underneath and collapsed in bitter tears.

By Saturday—the operation had been on a Thursday—she was busy organizing her three roommates. It was a multinational room, typically New York. There was a Jewish lady, named Ada something, in the corner by the window. There was a black lady, Josephine, across from her, and a Puerto Rican woman, partially paralyzed, next to her. And, of course, Gladys, who described herself as a "poor Irish girl from the Bronx," though she hadn't lived in the bombed-out Bronx in a decade, and whose beautiful home on a cul-de-sac in suburban New Jersey was anything but poverty-stricken.

"Stop tummeling already," said Ada, when Gladys got up, her two Jackson-Pratt drains knocking this way and that, and started redecorating the room. But Ada's face showed that she loved the sudden excitement. She was a sad case. Not very old, but without a close family member or friend in the world. She devised all kinds of excuses to stay in the hospital, because she dreaded going home to an empty apartment.

Josephine turned out to be a special friend. She worked for an electrical-supply company uptown, and she and Gladys had mutual acquaintances. This wasn't so unusual, because Gladys knew so many people that sometimes it seemed she could come up with mutual acquaintances with almost anyone in the city.

The Puerto Rican woman next to her was a problem. She had had some kind of stroke, and her tongue was partially paralyzed. She would try to talk to Gladys, and Gladys would try to answer back in Bronx street Spanish, although she was no linguist. The result was a bit pathetic and a bit comical. Even the woman's family members had trouble understanding her.

At night this woman became very demanding, constantly ringing for the nurses and then having great difficulty making her needs understood. After a few days, however, she couldn't find her night bell and Gladys believed that the nurses were hiding it from her so that she couldn't bother them. Since she didn't sleep well when she was away from home, Gladys left the curtain between their two beds half open at night, so that she could hear the Spanish woman stirring and bring her what she needed.

Her family was, of course, appreciative when they found out. "When you come to Brooklyn, you come to see us in Robles Street," they said.

"That's a *terrible* street," Gladys said, with her typical directness.

"You come stay with us and nobody give you trouble," said the woman's husband.

"Viva Zapata, then, I'll come," said Gladys, laughing.

The next morning Gladys looked in the mirror and was appalled at what she saw. She usually wore her hair coiffed up, neat as a pin. Now, however, her hair looked dirty and lay flat and straggly around her head—"like an olive," she complained to her roommates.

"So what are you going to do about it?" asked Ada. "You're in the hospital, so there's nothing to be done."

"We'll just see about that," said Gladys, getting that determined look on her face that usually spelled mischief. "There happens to be a beauty parlor right here on First Avenue. I passed it last time when I was coming in. I think I'm going to get me a perm."

"And how the hell are you going to get out of here?" asked Josephine skeptically.

"Simple," said Gladys, rising and getting her coat from the closet. With difficulty, she got it on.

"I'm going to walk right on out of here. And you people are going to be my alibi, understand? If that nurse comes in here, and wants to give me a shot or something, you just act very natural and tell her I've gone for a walk. It's true, too. You just don't have to say *where* I went for a walk."

She wrapped herself in her coat, covering her two telltale plastic drains, and proceeded to walk down the hallway, nodding to the nurse on duty. It looked as if she were going to the patients' lounge, but when she reached the end of the hallway, she glanced backward. The desk nurse was busy with some drug forms, and Gladys made a mad dash across the corridor and over to the bank of elevators. She got on a slow-going down elevator and, after an interminable ride, eventually found herself in the lobby of the building. She had learned years ago that if you wanted to fool people, you had to act like you knew exactly what you were doing. It was people's awkward behavior, nine times out of ten, that gave them away. And so she smiled at the square-badged guard, who smiled back, and jauntily made her way out onto the avenue.

In the beauty parlor there was a bit of a stir when this unkempt woman arrived in her slippers, and more of a stir when her coat fell open briefly to reveal two hanging plastic bags.

"May we help you?" asked the very neat fellow behind the counter.

"I'd like a perm or something. I'm sick and tired of looking like this."

"Well," said the man, eyeing her strangely. "I'm afraid you've come to the wrong place. First of all, you need an appointment. Second of all, we only do *natural* cutting here. We'll wash your hair and blow-dry it, but we only use hypoallergenic products and none of the harsh chemicals associated with permanents."

Gladys looked at him incredulously.

"What planet are you from?" she asked finally. "What am I asking for? You call yourself a beauty parlor—"

"A cutting emporium, to be exact," said the man.

"—and you can't even give me a perm." This was unheard of where she was from. "And here I come all the way from the hospital, get out of my death bed for you. Forget it. Forget it!"

The man was startled. "Are you really from Beth Israel? Do they know you're here?"

"What am I," said Gladys, "a kid out of school? If I feel like a perm, I'm going to get a perm. And what are you going to do, tell the teacher on me?"

The man looked away. Gladys strolled jauntily out of the cutting emporium and back across First Avenue, dodging traffic. She ignored the pain in her side. She walked through the entrance, on past the guards, and back up to her room.

Outside the elevator stood Ms. Dorothy McCardle, the head nurse, a niece of the surgeon McCardle and another one of Gladys's myriad social acquaintances.

"And where the hell were you?" said the nurse, a red-haired woman of imposing voice and dimensions. "I went down the front hall looking for you, Gladys. It's time for your bone scan."

"Oh, no," said Gladys levelly. "That's already been taken care of."

"What do you mean, 'taken care of'?" said McCardle, consulting her charts. "Yesterday you had the liver scan, right? Today's bone scan. I made the appointments myself."

"I can't hang around that long, though," said Gladys, resettling herself in the bed. She was panting—and wondered for a moment if she hadn't overdone it this time. "I got the boy to take me down yesterday afternoon for the bone scan. They said the dye would be out of my system. He was a nice kid. I told him, 'Don't worry about overtime. I'll pay you,' but he didn't take a dime. Nice kid."

Ordinarily McCardle would have been livid, but Gladys' manner was basically so innocent it was disarming.

"I give up," McCardle said, grumbling in a good-natured way. "You're really determined to get out of here, aren't you?" she said.

"You betcha," said Gladys. "Nothing personal," she added, "but I hate these places. It's no place for a sick person."

Dr. Strong had asked Gladys to "look down," look at herself, before leaving the hospital. This was a technique worked out after discussions with Dr. Lucas, the psychologist who served as consultant to the Breast Health Program. Sometimes a patient refused to look at herself after the operation, and that habit persisted even after she went home. The wound then became a festering psychological scar, more dangerous in its way than an infected physical scar. If they were going to have any untoward reaction, it would be better for it to happen in the hospital while Strong still had his eye on them.

Gladys showed no sign of following orders and so Strong asked Ms. McCardle to assist him. She gently reminded Gladys about it, a day before she was due to leave. "You've got to do it, Gladys. You can't avoid the topic entirely forever."

Gladys sat up in the bed. "What do I want to do that for? Look at the freak of nature? The half pint? The hung-low wonder?"

"It's for the best," said McCardle. "Do you want me to help you? I can remove the bandages."

"No, no," said Gladys, her essential vulnerability showing very quickly in her soft brown eyes and quavering voice.

McCardle drew the curtain, but stood in the hallway outside the door with an ear cocked for problems. Gladys gingerly removed the tape that held on the bandage. She gasped when she saw the top of the wound. There were staples in her—metal! Like most surgeons nowadays, after sewing up the incision with sutures, Strong then used staples to hold the wound together.

Christ, she thought, I'll get electrocuted if there's ever a thunderstorm. I'm like the tin man in *The Wizard of Oz*.

She pulled the bandage off further and a small cry emerged from her throat. It was gone. All her delusions, her laughing denials and dismissals suddenly evaporated, leaving her with a massive kind of emptiness. She sobbed, but not as loudly or bitterly as she had thought she would. So this was it. That's all. A nothing. It's so—*disgusting!* So unbalanced. She felt violated, mutilated, crippled. Nothing would ever make this better, no amount of counseling or visits from well-wishers or volunteers or pep talks would ever bring back her precious breast. She had been so proud of them all her life, she was so well endowed, they were something to guard jealously from predatory males; yet that was half the fun in life—showing them off, swinging her equally well-endowed behind, going around to the plumbing factories and the wholesalers and flirting with the guys—and now all that was gone. They might not know—but of course they would know! They'd look down on her and their eyes would focus knowingly on something lacking there, something stiff and unnatural, or a bit crooked. The jokes would spread, for eventually everybody joined in the jokes about that kind of thing. She had made some herself back in the old days, before she was the object of jokes or worse, of pity.

She thought of the women she had known who had had this same operation. She couldn't believe it, that they had really gone through this hell. And what about her husband? What about sex? What now? She would never let him see this. No one would see this. When she would take a shower—and how she longed to take a shower, something forbidden to the post-mastectomy hospital patient—she would make sure to lock the door. She had never been big on nudity, but now even her daughter would not be allowed to see. Forget it!

"Are you all right, dear?" asked a voice from outside the curtain. Gladys pulled the cover over herself, a look of panic on her face. It was only Dotty McCardle.

"Yeah, I'm okay," said Gladys, her voice instantly betraying her, as it often did.

"Would you like some help in putting it back?"

"Nothing will put it back," she said bitterly. McCardle drew the curtain and could see the tear stains and the ashen complexion.

"You won't believe me," the nurse said gently, sitting down on the edge of the bed and speaking low so the roommates couldn't hear. "But this too will pass. This feeling. You came to identify that breast with *you*. But you'll get used to the new you. And after all, think of it this way. It could have been an arm or a leg, right? Imagine walking around with a hook—" she held out her arm grotesquely "—or a peg leg. You'd hobble around like Long John Silver."

Gladys laughed faintly, but more to be polite than anything. She knew differently. Nothing would ever be the same again.

In the weeks that followed, everything might have returned more or less to normal for Gladys, if it hadn't been for the chemotherapy. At least her hair hadn't fallen out, hadn't even thinned, and for that she could be grateful. But otherwise she hated the treatment.

When Strong had suggested drugs—based on the size of her tumor and the fact that at least one of her nodes was positive for cancer—she had shuddered. She, like most people, had heard about the side effects of cancer chemotherapy.

"Give me the top and the bottom line," she had said to him.

"Well, if you want to live, you'll take it," said Strong. "Survival figures are better for women like yourself who get chemotherapy than for those who don't."

"And what happens if I don't take it?" she said, in that stubborn and independent way of hers.

"No one can say," said Strong. "It just improves the odds quite a bit."

She thought it over and took it.

The pills were harder for her than the injections. She just couldn't seem to get them down. All her life she had rejected medicine and said she would die before even taking an aspirin. The Cytoxan pills would simply stick in her throat. She kept a sixteen-ounce glass by the sink precisely for this purpose, but it didn't help. No matter how much water she took with them, they seemed to stick.

It was difficult, if not impossible, to describe to Sam the feelings she got from the medicine. Her mouth tasted like ashes. She would get nauseated, but it was more like the nausea you get during a hangover—just a rotten feeling in which food is a particularly disgusting thought. She would sweat around the neck even when others were cold. Other things started to go wrong. Her eyes began to burn. She asked Dr. Vogel if the Cytoxan could do that, if they could affect the eyes to the point that they began to tear. And he said, yes, photophobia was one of the side effects of the drug. There were many others, and one day she was alarmed to read a description of them all in the *Physicians Desk Reference* she found in a Paramus Mall bookstore. She almost stopped taking the pills right then and there. She also read that some people only had to take the chemotherapy for six months, and she was suspicious of the doctors' motives in telling her to take it for a full year.

"Don't be a wisenheimer," Sam told her. "Take the medicine like they tell you."

It was easy for him to say, of course; he didn't have to put up with the rotten feeling, nor with the terrible loss of energy that made so many days such an interminable drag.

Well, this was her "Knute Rockne" bit, as she called it. Eventually she would get her first down, if not her touchdown. Time simply went by and soon it would be over.

Gladys was very self-conscious about her looks. She studied herself in the full-length mirror in the hall. It's hard to grow old under any circumstances, but she would catch frightening glimpses of a strange middle-aged person staring back at her from the mirror. Her mind would reject this quickly and replace it with a more pleasing picture. And, in fact, if she smiled, or practiced a seductive look in the mirror, she could again see the bright, cheerful, sexy Gladys of Bronx days.

The most important change was a subtle one: cancer had become part of her. She noticed it everywhere, and her heart went out to the people who were its victims. She read the obituary page with a strange fascination and felt a kinship with the people dying of cancer or those who "succumbed after a long illness." She read books about it, studied them, pencil in hand, whereas until then her main reading material had been the *Star-Ledger* and trashy novels. Sam teased her. "What are you, going into the cancer business?"

Gladys went back to work and eventually everybody either forgot about that stiff falsie on her breast or just ran out of things to say.

One day a customer called and sounded funny. "Mr. Dooley," she said, "you don't sound yourself." She thought maybe he had "half a bag on," a condition not unusual in some of her customers after a long bar lunch.

"No, Gladys," he whispered hoarsely. "I've got cancer."

The revelation electrified her—the more so when she suddenly realized, I've got it, too. I've got cancer, too, Mr. Dooley. But she didn't say that. She only said, "I'm awfully sorry to hear that."

"Yes, I've got cancer of the larynx," he said. He pronounced it "larnex." "I've had a larnexectomy."

She felt bad—she had thought he was drunk, probably everyone else did too, when actually the poor man had had his voice box removed. He was probably speaking with one of those synthetic voice-makers they press to their throats. Gladys was tempted to tell him about herself, but hesitated. Somehow she didn't want to be associated with this pathetic-sounding man.

"I'm sorry to hear that, Mr. Dooley. Sorry I don't have time to talk now. Make sure you come in and see me when you're next in the shop."

She went into the cramped ladies' room and stared at herself in the mirror. Her eyes were tearing, but she wasn't sure whether that was caused by her pity for Mr. Dooley or just the effects of the drug.

Mildred

Mildred's mastectomy went off without a hitch. Strong did a "transverse incision"—a low, sideways cut rather than the old standard incision that came diagonally across the breast. The transverse looked better and was better for reconstructive surgery. Because of the extent of the disease in Mildred's case, however, reconstruction was not advisable for a year or two. Also, she would require radiotherapy, and this would make the skin a bit thicker and more difficult for the plastic surgeon to work with.

The mastectomy involved removing all the lymph nodes under the arm, but not the nerves or the muscles in that region. A minimal amount of swelling would always be present, because the lymph nodes of the armpit normally drained fluid from the arm. And Mildred would have to be careful to avoid fingernail infections in that hand and not to allow blood to be taken from that arm. The lymph system protected against infection and with the nodes gone she was at greater risk of developing an infection in that area.

During the operation Strong found that the tumor involved the central quadrant and the inner quadrant of the breast, near the sternum. It became obvious that, as he had suspected, radiotherapy to these areas would become necessary to maintain good loco-regional control of the tumor.

After the operation, they wheeled Mildred into the recovery room. Slowly consciousness came back to her. Her first sensation was one of overwhelming nausea. She wretched piteously into a kidney-shaped dish provided by one of the nurses.

Her next thought was of her teeth.

"I want my teeth," she mumbled. She wore dentures, but naturally they had been taken from her before the operation. She had made the nurses promise they would give them back to her immediately after the surgery.

"When you get up to your room," said the recovery-room nurse.

Mildred felt betrayed, but she was too sick and exhausted to argue. Later she was to reflect on the peculiarity of human nature; here she was, sick as a dog, having just lost a breast, but worrying about someone seeing her without her dentures!

The day passed in a vague sort of way. She remembered seeing her son's and daughter's faces, but they disappeared into the same fog into which everything evaporated. Philip came by —poor Phil, who was so afraid of doctors that he had run out of the room at his own son's circumcision! What a trial it was for him, she could see by his face. She held his hand, she remembered that, but then he too was gone.

Slowly she emerged from this trauma, but as she did, she became aware that another trauma was waiting for her. Dr. Kurz came by: he had been sent by Dr. Strong, he said, to check up on her. When her own physician had retired to Florida, she had been left without a family doctor of her own. Kurz checked her bandages and asked her how she was feeling in a gentle voice.

"How should I be feeling?" she whispered. "Like dancing at Roseland?"

The next thing she knew it was morning and Leslie Strong was sitting by her bed. "How are you doing, Mildred?"

"I feel a lot better," she said hoarsely.

"You *look* a lot better," he said. "I looked in on you last night. You've gotten most of your color back."

"This was no piece of cake," she said.

"I never said it was going to be easy," said Strong.

"I mean, I had a partial hysterectomy, I had a thyroid tumor, but they were *nothing* compared to this. Nothing."

Almost involuntarily her hand went to her breast. There was a big, bulky bandage there, but she could feel the emptiness underneath and her heart sank. No matter how many times she had told herself that this was inevitable, no matter how many times Strong explained to her, it was still hard to believe.

Strong sat there silently. This was the moment he always dreaded the most.

"So tell me," she said finally.

"Of course you know. We had to remove the breast. You've had a modified radical mastectomy."

She looked at him, and, despite all the mental preparations, it was still a shock.

"There wasn't any way to save . . . ?"

"We took as little as we could," he said gently. "But—I have to tell you this, dear—the lymph nodes *were* involved. I took out twenty-four of them, and seventeen of them had cancer."

"Seventeen?" she said uncomprehendingly.

"That's very advanced, Mildred."

She now realized what that meant. "I'm so stupid," she said. "I let this thing go for God knows how long and all the while it was growing, spreading. Do you think if I had come right away, it might not have spread so?"

"Perhaps. It really all depends on the 'cell kinetics,'" said Strong. "The way the tumor develops over time. You see, Mildred, before a breast cancer becomes palpable it must be about two centimeters in diameter—about the size of a pea. But to reach that stage takes between seven and ten *years,* in the average case.

"In general the earlier the tumor is found, the greater the disease-free period of survival, and the more possibilities of surgical alternatives.

"So, it's not great news," he said finally, "but we knew that, right? We'll deal with it the best we can. You're going to need further treatment to get at the cancer cells that could not be treated surgically. The good news is that we got the results of the bone scans, liver scan, and the CEA levels, which is a kind of chemical marker for cancer present in the body. They're all normal. We can't find any evidence of other tumors in your body, at least with the technology that's available to us today. But we have a good supposition that there are still some small colonies of cells, micrometastases, as they're called, somewhere else in your body. That's because of the size and extent and aggressiveness of your tumor. And that's why you're going to need further treatment, to try and destroy those tiny nests of cells."

"What do you mean 'try?'" Mildred asked. "Let's go in there and get them!"

"You're terrific," Strong said, and he meant it. "I wish I had a hundred patients like you!"

She looked at him steadily. "Yeah? I wish you had none!"

So far, she had been so occupied with tests, procedures, conversations about the future, visits of relatives bearing fruit and flowers, that she hadn't had a moment's peace. She knocked around the floor with her two drainage sacks—what she called her "Harvey Wallbangers"—sticking out.

On a late afternoon, two days before going home, she found that moment. She was alone in the room. Her roommate with Alzheimer's Disease had been taken down for some more tests, and her hired aide had gone with her. It was a rough and windy autumn day outside, the sky a bruised color, with an aura of anticipation over the city. She pulled the curtain around her bed.

Of course, they had come to change her bandages: she had turned away, hadn't looked. But you couldn't go through life like this, although she had heard that some people did. Molly had told her about a case—someone she knew through Cancer Care—who had vowed never to look at herself after her mastectomy. For eight years this woman had gone along, never opening her eyes in the bathtub, keeping herself covered, avoiding mirrors. *Meshugah!* Crazy! She couldn't live like that. Yet in a strange way she could feel the temptation, the allure of it. Just *refuse* to deal with the terrible fact. I will not accept this loss of a breast! If I don't look at it, it never happened, and I am back to normal again, instead of a freak.

No, that way madness lies, the rational part of her argued loudly. You can't live your life—however many years are left to you—like a recluse, a hermit.

And so she opened the beautiful rayon nightgown Phil had brought her—all baby pinks and blues—and looked. Her right breast looked the same: still beautiful to her and her husband. An object of sexual power, of sexual identity. But where the left breast had been—nothing. Nothing!

She closed the gown, a look of amazed horror on her face,

her mouth open in a circle. Where had it gone? How could this be possible? Her very identity, her sense of Mildred, had been violated.

For her breasts were *her*, in a deep sense. This was not just a piece of clothing she could discard. Now, suddenly, instead of her beautiful bubby, there was nothing but a bandage, with a couple of hideous tubes sticking out of it.

She felt a sudden surge of anger, of rage, toward Dr. Strong, toward her husband, toward the whole frigging male world, the male conspiracy that had deprived her of her breast. This just couldn't be. She could never accept this.

She placed her hand over the bandage, and slowly felt the flatness of it. She was like a little girl again, she mused, and the thought was somehow consoling. Yes, you could think about it that way: before she was thirteen, she had been flat-chested, but she had still been Milly. And she could, therefore, be without her breasts again and still be Milly. *She* was not *her breasts*. She was more than them, more than any particular part of her body.

Slowly, uncertainly, she lifted the strips of adhesive and looked underneath. There was a long wound where her breast had been. It was a good clean line, she noted. Strong had done a good job. It was wrong to be mad at him. He was only doing his job, the best he could do. And he hadn't done anything she hadn't agreed to have him do.

But it wasn't his breast. He wouldn't have to live with this for the rest of his life. To confront this every morning, this mutilation, this lopsidedness, this fear.

She suddenly had that special feeling we all occasionally have—that we have arrived at a crossroads in life, a moment of internal, mental decision. Having the operation was not the crossroads: that was a gross physical fact. The crossroads were *now*, this very instant, and she saw it plainly in her mind, without words, in a kind of mental picture. She could either go the way of rejection—of retreat deeper and deeper into herself—or acceptance, of the terrible reality that life or fate had presented to her.

She chose life. Later on, of course, everyone would say, "Mildred is making a wonderful recovery," as if that recovery just came automatically. Cheerful Milly, bright Milly, the Milly you could always count on. But she knew that it was her choice, and that it had come through a struggle. She had stood at the abyss of despair and pulled back. She would go on.

Radiation, chemotherapy—they would throw it all at her and she would survive. Because she had something to live for, not just life itself, but the wonderful people whom she had managed to surround herself with. How terrible for those other women—the majority, she thought—who never knew the love of a really fine and devoted man like Philip, or the wonderful feeling—the *nachas,* or joy—of seeing their children grow up into fine adults, loving, devoted, and caring. For them alone, it would be worth surviving.

Who the hell cares about a titty? As Phil said, he can love the other one twice as much. She knew that they would pick up the pieces, their life would go on, even their love life would go on. Maybe better than ever, because they would have proven their love even more through this trial.

Her thoughts were interrupted suddenly as the curtain was pulled back.

It was the Jamaican nurse, a newfound friend.

"How are you, Mrs. Rosenbloom?" she asked, in that wonderful accent.

"Me?" said Mildred, laughing. "Couldn't be better."

Gladys

Some time later, Gladys got a visit at work from George Stack. He was one of the salesmen from Navesink Plumbing whom she had known for ages. When her first husband was alive they had loved to socialize with George and Eileen. She and Eileen, in fact, had almost gone into politics together in the Bronx; they had been active in the PTA, the Kiwanis, the Rotary Club.

She hadn't heard from George and Eileen in a long time, although it was always in the back of her mind to give them a call. Now, in a sense, it was her operation that held her back. Not only had it taken up her time, while also taking away much of her energy, but she just didn't feel like explaining again what had happened. She was still ashamed of it in a way. She was afraid she would seem somehow diminished in their eyes.

"What's happening, George? Since you changed territories I don't get to see you anymore."

"Yeah," he said uncomfortably, "it's a pity. I miss the old times." Something else was clearly on his mind, but Gladys was giving him time to get to his point.

"How's Eileen? God, sometimes I miss that tough old dame."

George laughed—sort of snorted—sardonically. "Some tough old dame," he mumbled.

"Why? What's the matter?" Gladys said, immediately alarmed.

"You wouldn't recognize her," said George, and she could sense the real concern in his voice.

"What's wrong?"

"Hell, Gladys, I can't talk about it now." He lowered his voice. "Maybe we could get together for a drink sometime?"

"What's wrong with now?"

"Is it okay?" he asked dubiously.

"It's slow this morning," she said. "Come on, I'll treat you to one."

They went around the corner to the Blarney Stone, with its friendly smells of beer and the corned beef and cabbage being readied for the noontime crush.

When they were settled in—George with his scotch and soda, Gladys with a Lite beer—he started to pour out his troubles.

"Listen, Gladys, I'd be lying if I said I didn't know about your problem." He unconsciously glanced at her breasts.

"How'd you find out?" she asked, trying to sound unemotional. She'd like to fix the rat who was going around spreading rumors about her.

"What does it matter?" he asked. "The point is, I can sympathize with what you're going through because me and Eileen have been through the ringer on this for the last few years."

"You have?" said Gladys, amazed. "You mean she—"

"Two years ago. Up there at Misericordia. Took it off." He was speaking low. "But the worst goddamn thing is—I mean, you're going about your business, functioning, like nothing happened—" Gladys laughed. "—but Eileen's become a recluse—" He emphasized the second syllable. "—who don't want to go out, don't want to see nobody, or socialize, or nothing. I mean, you wouldn't recognize her today, Gladys. You wouldn't believe it was the Eileen of old."

"Oh, George, that's terrible," she said.

"I wouldn't drag you into this, except I think maybe you can help me, and I'm desperate. You know—" He lowered his voice again, which had been gaining in volume as he got into his problem. "—I haven't slept in my own bed in two years." He gave her a meaningful glance, and took a gulp of his drink. "I and Eileen, we—well, haven't you know, been man and wife, since this happened. I mean, the scar don't mean shit to me, and that's Gospel, but as far as she's concerned, it's all over. You get my meaning?"

Too well, thought Gladys, but she just nodded.

"And now she thinks I've got another woman tucked away somewhere."

"No one could blame you if you did," Gladys said softly.

"But that's the damn thing. I don't. I don't want no one but Eileen. But she just drives me away. So I don't hurry to get home, if you know what I mean. I just take my time about it. Make the round of the bars, stay a little longer each time, have an extra belt or two. It's bad, Gladys. I'm falling into a trap. I know it. And then my brother's got a boat—he's a bachelor, you remember—and so on the weekend I like to go out fishing with him. She thinks I'm with my girlfriend," he said, laughing at the absurdity of the situation.

"What do you want me to do?" Gladys asked.

"Could you maybe go talk to her? I mean, if anybody could, you could. I better warn you, though, it won't be easy. She's one goddamn stubborn woman, but if anyone can get through to her, maybe you can."

On Saturday, Gladys packed a little duffel bag full of special items and drove up to the Bronx. The Stacks had a narrow two-story house with a wraparound sun porch and two back doors—one of them was the "service" entrance when the house was built, around the turn of the century. That was the door Gladys went to, as she always had in the days when she and Eileen were best of friends.

She rang the bell, but there was no answer. Somehow she didn't think Eileen was out, not after what George had told her. She rang again, and then rapped on the window. She could have sworn she saw something stirring behind the curtain, but then it disappeared.

Gladys placed the gym bag she had brought with her on the ground. She pushed hard, opened the kitchen window a couple of inches, and yelled in, "Hey, Eileen, you ain't fooling me. I know you're in there."

There was silence and then a voice tentatively answered, "Who's that? Is that you, Gladys?"

"So who the hell did you think it was? Santa Claus?"

There was a scurrying inside. Meanwhile Gladys removed several items from her bag and put them on. By the time Eileen opened the door a crack, Gladys was standing there with a stethoscope in her ears and a blood pressure cuff on her arm. These items were leftovers from the days when her first husband was on the dialysis machine. She had also dressed in official-looking black slacks and a white blouse, and had even borrowed a green medical jacket. It was a credible imitation of a visiting doctor.

Eileen took one look at her and started laughing—for the first time in months, or maybe even years.

"You always was a character," she said.

"Can I come in?" Gladys said, literally putting her foot in the door.

"Do I have any choice in the matter?" said Eileen. "Jeez, I look a wreck. I hate to have you see me like this. Did George tell you to do this?" Her voice was suddenly suspicious.

"You crazy old dame," said Gladys, artfully dodging the question. "You think he gives a damn about you anymore, what with the way you're treating him. Sure I saw him at the store, but comin' here was my own idea. Plus I got something else to show you."

They went into the kitchen. Gladys remembered in the old days when it was neat and clean, when there was always something good cooking on the stove. Now it was depressing. The garbage was piled up in grocery bags. There was a bad odor coming from the sink, and there was grunge everywhere.

Seeing Eileen herself was also painful. She had aged terribly. Of course, they had all aged, but at least Gladys had kept herself up. She still felt good enough about herself, in fact, to have a pastel portrait done when they were up at a Catskills resort the month after the operation and to hang it over her mantelpiece. But Eileen had bags under her eyes and had let her hair grow out gray and unkempt. It was a pitiful sight to anyone who knew her in the old days, when she and Gladys had led the protest for school crossing guards.

"What did you mean with that crack about George? What's he been telling you? I bet he didn't tell you he's got another broad stashed away somewhere."

"That's bunk, Eileen," Gladys said vehemently. "He ain't

got no girl anywhere. He's off getting soused every night and you're too dumb to realize it." To an outsider it would have sounded very harsh, but they had always talked in this playfully rough way with each other, and Eileen loved and understood it.

"You think so?" she asked.

"Not that I would blame him if he did have a piece somewhere. Christ, the poor guy hasn't had any in years."

"You don't understand," said Eileen, sagging down at the kitchen table. She had put up water for coffee, although in truth Gladys didn't look forward to drinking from her soiled cups. "Did he tell you . . . why?"

They had clearly entered the painful part of the conversation, but Gladys had made up her mind to tough it through.

"You mean about your—" She was about to say something gross, but decided to cool it. "—breast operation?"

"So he's going around telling everyone now?"

"Cut it, Eileen. You and I go back. He had to tell somebody, and so he told me."

"Well, so you know. Next thing you're gonna want is a free show. A look at the freak. That's why I keep the lights so low in here. That way *nobody* can see, not even me. To tell you the truth, hon, I've never even looked at it. Never. And I never intend to."

Eileen poured the coffee—luckily she had disposable hot cups to pour it into—and leaned back. Gladys could see the unnatural bulge beneath the torn nightgown. (Goddamn it, she thought, she's probably using a rolled-up pair of socks in her bra, like when we were kids.)

"I'm glad you came, but where the hell were you when I needed you?"

Gladys had her opening. "Where was I? I was in the hospital having the same thing done to me that they done to you. What do you think?"

Why was it so enjoyable to pull surprises on people like this? She didn't know, but she relished the expression of shock, amazement, and then compassion that came over Eileen's face.

Now they were no longer just friends—they were also comrades.

"Are you kidding?" she finally whispered.

"Wanna see my scars? I'll show you mine if you show me yours," said Gladys, with a bravado she hardly felt.

"When?"

"Just a few months ago. Plus I'm on chemotherapy, which is no picnic. But I don't let it ruin my life. I may croak tomorrow. The cancer may come back or I may get hit by a semi, walking out of here. I don't know. All I know is I intend to enjoy life while I've got it. It's the only life I've got or am likely to get for a long while."

As Eileen poured a second cup of coffee, Gladys said, "You know, I've been giving this a lot of thought. It seems to me that when you discover a lump you've got basically four decisions to make, four choices. First, of course, you go into a panic, but that wears off and then comes decision time."

"For me, there weren't any choices," said Eileen. "I just did what I was told."

"That's what I'm talking about," Gladys said, emphatically. "That's probably why you feel so miserable. You feel like you let your life slip out of control. But in reality you did make the first decision, and that was whether or not to go to a doctor."

"That's a decision?"

"You bet it is! You know me, hon, I can't stand doctors. Never could. I put it off for the longest time and if it hadn't been for my daughter maybe I still wouldn't have gone. But that first choice can mean your life.

"The next big choice is, 'Do I surrender to the doctor or do I make the big decisions for myself?'"

"I was never offered that choice," said Eileen. "They just—"

"Bull," said Gladys. "The choice was yours, but you just didn't want to face it. This is a free country and no doctor can decide for you what's going to be done with your body.

"The third choice you have to make is what kind of treatment to have. It used to be simple. Mastectomy. But now things have changed and there's a whole smorgasbord of choices. Or maybe you don't want any treatment at all. The choice is yours."

"I guess you're right," said Eileen, quietly. "But I just wasn't brought up to think this way. To make these kinds of decisions. Anyway, that's all behind me now, water over the dam. Maybe I was a jerk, but I let them do what they had to do and that was the end of that."

"Which brings me to my final choice," said Gladys. She had rehearsed this little speech in her mind before coming over, but it was something to which she had given a great deal of thought, working it out in those hours between the time she awoke and she actually got out of bed in the morning. "This one definitely concerns you, dear, because it's the choice you haven't made yet."

"And what's that?" asked Eileen, obviously intrigued.

"Whether to go on living," said Gladys.

"That's a question?"

"Yes, it is. What I mean is, How are you going to live the rest of your life? Like a hermit crab or like a real, live person? Okay, so you lost a goddamned breast. Are you going to let that stop you from living life to the fullest?"

Eileen sighed again, but this time not quite so deeply. Gladys felt that her words were starting to have an effect.

"Look, I know it's a big thing," Gladys said, more softly now. "But it's a fact, right? You accept it and then you get on with your business. You've got to make that fourth choice. I mean, lookit, you've got a husband who's sleeping on the sofa, and why? Not because he doesn't find you attractive, but because you haven't made up your mind yet whether you're going to live or die." She paused. "Okay, end of sermon. But I brought you something to sort of illustrate the lecture. I wasn't sure if I was gonna give you this, but now I see it's very appropriate. I was afraid you'd misconstrue it." She removed a big balloon from her bag, the kind street peddlers sell on 34th Street, and started to blow it up. She got it about half blown up when she ran out of breath, but it was already almost three feet tall, with a ridiculous clown's face in three colors.

"What the hell are you doing, you maniac?" Eileen screamed with delight. "You always was a maniac." She punched Gladys in the arm, which made her laugh and lose some of the air in a rush of obscene noise. They both giggled, but Gladys got the balloon under control again and tied it off.

"Okay, hold this. Now I also brought you these."

She reached into her bag of tricks and pulled out a lily she had picked up that morning on her way to the Bronx and a wooden yard ruler she had taken from work.

"What the hell is all this? So tell me."

"Okay. I brought the ruler to measure your coffin and the lily to put in your hands." She folded her hands over her chest.

"That's the one way. Or you can have the balloon. It's your choice. Take your pick, but it's got to be one or the other."

Eileen laughed heartily, her old belly laugh, and Gladys thought: hey, this is really going to work! She repeated her line about the lily and the ruler a few times. She had thought of that the night before—it was an inspiration.

Eileen reached over and hugged Gladys around the neck. She could feel the tears on her cheek.

"I've been acting crazy, haven't I?" said Eileen. "I mean, it's true, I've been putting George through the ropes and blaming him, when it's not his fault. It's just been so hard. . . . I didn't know anyone, have anyone to talk to or to understand."

"You should have called me," said Gladys, although she could understand very well the emotion her friend was describing.

"I was so ashamed. I felt like no one would want me, that I was tainted, useless, like an old shoe."

"Well, that's a crock. Starting today, you're gonna pull yourself together. There's thousands of women like us out there. Millions, probably. Maybe you and me, we'll get them all together, get them fighting together for better treatment and what not. Just like the old days."

"You're a born politician," said Eileen.

"You're another one," said Gladys. "First thing is, we've got to get this mess cleaned up."

"No, to be honest, the first thing is for me to get some kind of—what do you call it?—prosthetic device. I've been ashamed to go out because I look so terrible, so *obvious*. I need to get to a store that sells them, but I don't know where to start. Do you think maybe you could drive me downtown?"

Gladys smiled. "Hey, what the hell do you think friends are for?"

Robin

There is a whole subculture of dog owners in Manhattan, and Robin was part of it. First you get to know the pooch, then you get to know the owner, although the masters rarely goi as intimate as the dogs—or at least not quite as fast.

Robin's apartment was within walking distance of Central Park, and in the morning, which, when she was waitressing, began around noon, she liked to go over to the Metropolitan Museum and then stroll down to the open meadows. Her ancient wirehair, Barney, trotted alongside her She carried a piece of newspaper in her hand for Barney's inevitable donation.

It was a lovely late autumn day. She strolled past the steps of the museum and then had a moment of panic. All these horse-faced preppies on the steps of the Metropolitan were laughing, and she had the very real sensation that they were laughing at her.

She stopped, turned around, saw nothing, and continued to walk. The laughter became more uproarious. With a red face, she suddenly realized what it was. She wheeled around unexpectedly and caught a mime, his face painted death-mask white, prancing behind her, mimicking her galumphing walk. A few tourists, from the safety of the steps, snapped pictures. Native New Yorkers snickered knowingly.

Her first impulse was to smack him. But his mimicry was so exact, and therefore so funny, that she decided there was no real reason to be angry. Besides, she would look an even greater fool if she showed her anger. So she took his arm and strolled along with him, trying to mimic *him* and doing a pretty good job of it. At least the impromptu crowd roard with appreciation.

Into the park, past the new American wing, she went on down the path. She kicked the fallen leaves in front of her as she walked, the way she used to do when she was a kid. It was good to be alive on days like this. If only it wasn't for this frigging chemotherapy, she could enjoy her life . . . day by day. But she felt so bad all the time, so exhausted beyond words. If only she could give it up. The idea had occurred to her more than once, but then she wondered: won't I feel like a fool if the cancer comes back? I mean, what's the use of doing it for so many months only to give up before the race is finished?

Along the path came another wirehair, whom Barney recognized as an old friend, Sam. She thought of that quip she had read in *Time* magazine: dogs can laugh, but they do it with their tails. Barney also laughed with his mouth: a silent, somewhat foolish, slobbering grin. The two dogs circled each other inquisitively. Sam was a female—Samantha, Robin guessed, or else named by a person with a poor grasp of anatomy.

Behind Sam came her master, a guy she knew only as Mark. Mark was jogging along in his matching sweatsuit, looking healthy and exhausted. A patch of wetness dampened his chest like a badge of merit. He stopped when he saw Robin and gave her a big hello. He was good-looking, in a funny way. He had a big black mustache and big black eyebrows that gave him a comical look.

"Robin, how you doing?" he panted, laughing. He took her hand affectionately.

"I'm all right," she said, in the way of sick people who really want to tell their story but at the same time don't want to complain.

"Haven't seen you in a long time," Mark pursued. "Want to go for a little walk?"

"It looks like we're doing that," she said.

They both laughed. "So what's new with you? What are you up to?"

"I'm just taking Barney out to do his duty," she said. "Then I thought I'd head over to the drugstore and see if my pictures are ready. I found this old roll and thought I'd have it developed."

"Chemists. Drugstores are only drugstores in the boroughs. In Manhattan they become pharmacies. And then, on the East Side between, say, 34th Street and 96th Street, they become chemists. Don't ask me why."

She laughed happily. "You're a riot. It's true. God, this place drives me crazy sometimes, it's so phoney. You know, the Greek coffee shop around my way is now called a twenty-four-hour cocktail lounge. They've got one of these arty neon signs that must have cost them about ten thousand dollars. Then there's David's Cookies, haberdashers—"

"Don't forget stationers—"

"Apothecaries, that's another one. One step up from chemists, in fact. God, that's a riot." She hadn't laughed like this in a long time. It felt good.

"So where have you been?" Mark said, sounding almost artificially nonchalant.

"Well, I've been sick," she admitted. "I was in the hospital for a while, and I've been on some heavy-duty medicine. So I haven't felt like going out much. I just take Barney here outside the building, then go back upstairs."

There was a pause.

"Robin, do you mind if I get a bit personal?" She waited, not saying anything. "I'm pretty familiar with this whole business, if you know what I mean."

"No, I don't know what you mean," she said, almost hostile.

"Cancer, Robin." She started to object, for reasons she couldn't yet fathom, but he silenced her. "Listen to me, hon. I know what you're going through . . . but if you just hang in there and *use your head,* you're gonna be okay."

"How did you know?" asked Robin, just getting over the shock.

"Well, as I said, I'm pretty savvy on this topic. The hair, for one thing. Don't take offense, please. But I know what chemotherapy does to a person. Not that you look bad. Not at all. You're quite gorgeous. But, well, to an experienced eye . . ."

"I see," said Robin. No matter what he said, she was

shocked that it was so obvious. She wasn't ashamed of it . . . but she also didn't want people to notice. "I thank you for your opinions, Mark, but actually I don't think you *can* know what I'm going through. I mean healthy people like yourself—"

She went on, but Mark cracked up laughing in such a spontaneous way that she had to smile, too, although she didn't know exactly what the joke was.

"Yeah, I'm very healthy. I also, technically speaking, have terminal cancer."

"You what?"

"That's right, hon! According to my doctors, I am terminally ill with lung cancer. Oat-cell carcinoma, it's called. One of the worst types of disease there is."

"I—I can't believe this!"

"It's true. The next thing you're going to ask me is what's my secret remedy, right? Well, I don't really have any secrets. I was on chemotherapy myself, but after the second injection, I freaked out. God, I felt like death warmed over. I thought to myself: if I'm going to die, let me die with a little dignity, not like a dog puking my guts out on the bathroom floor!"

His words sounded a chord inside her. She knew the feeling, exactly.

"So you did what?" she asked eagerly.

"I had heard about a man, a doctor, who cured himself of cancer through diet and nutrition and so forth. I cut out the chemotherapy and called this man and started on his regimen. And, God, I felt a thousand times better. Like a new person. I gained weight—I had been down below a hundred pounds—and my hair grew back in, and I just feel terrific. I started meditating and exercising, as you can see."

"That's terrific." She couldn't believe what she was hearing. For a moment she felt like she was having a religious revelation, like she had come through the woods and glimpsed some great vista of which she had previously been unaware. It was a breathtaking thought. "And are you cured now?"

Mark hesitated. "Well, not exactly. I was okay for almost two years, but the last time I went to the physician there was another spot on my lung. A metastasis, they think. Also a dark area in my liver. They wanted to put me back on chemo, but I refused. I think I can live like this, Robin, I really do. You see,

I had run out of money, so I curtailed most of the vitamins and enzymes and minerals. They get pretty expensive, especially when you're not working. And I got kind of lazy about my health, complacent—although I didn't go so far as to start smoking again. Smoking had been my downfall. So now I'm running, twenty miles a day, believe it or not, and I'm back on the health diet, and I'm taking as many pills as possible. Come up to my house, and I'll show you everything I take. You won't believe it."

"Maybe some time," said Robin, wondering in the back of her mind if this was some kind of weird proposition.

"But here I am running on at the mouth. You haven't told me about you. What's your problem?"

"Breast," she said self-consciously. It was such a turnoff to so many guys that she hesitated to mention it, even though she and Peter were for all intents and purposes married and monogamous.

"Radical mastectomy?"

"Well, I had a modified radical mastectomy," she said. "I've got a very good doctor."

"That's terrific," he said, although she could tell that he didn't really mean it. He really disapproved of surgery, she could tell that, although he probably had scars enough of his own.

They had walked the path till they were at the exit of the park. "Listen, I've got to get over to the chemists or the apothecary or whatever they call it before they close. I'd like to hear the rest of your story. . . ."

"I'd be happy to accompany you, if you don't mind," he said sweetly. "Just let me get ol' Sam on a leash. She's terrified of traffic."

They walked down 72nd Street, in the direction of Leslie Strong's office, as a matter of fact. It was a small world, or at least a small island, with plenty of reminders of her condition if she was looking for them.

"You know I'm sorry I didn't run into you *last* week," Mark said. "We had a meeting here in New York, at the Roosevelt."

"We?" asked Robin. She was suspicious of such "we's."

"The health federation," said Mark. "There were over three thousand people here at our health jamboree. You would have loved it. Everything under the sun, everything you can imagine. There were plenty of people like yourself there, too. *Former* cancer victims."

"Are they all as healthy-looking as you?" Robin asked a bit sarcastically.

"Not all. They come too late. After surgery, radiation, and chemotherapy has wrecked their immune systems."

"That's a cheerful thought," said Robin. She was feeling so low these days, however, that she felt like a wreck.

"Well, it's true," Mark said earnestly. "You really should look into the *natural* way of controlling cancer. A healthy low-fat diet. Plenty of vitamins. ACE the cancer with A, C, and E. Fresh fruits and vegetables. And some of the non-toxic therapies."

"Well, what's done is done," said Robin; involuntarily she ran her hand over her thinning hair.

"Chemo is the pits," he said, as they reached the store where Robin's pictures were waiting. "Pure poison. It's no magic bullet, Robin. It can't distinguish between the good cells and the bad cells. That's why you feel so shitty all the time."

It was true, of course. No one, not even Dr. Vogel, she thought, would deny that. But the statistics showed that it did some good, too. Especially in cases like hers—pre-menopausal women with lymph node involvement—her new self-image. Up the odds of survival. In her case, the chances of recurrence were high and she needed all the breaks she could get. But what Mark said was deeply disturbing to her. She knew on an intellectual level that the man was probably something of a fanatic—nice, but one-sided in his judgment of modern medicine. But on an emotional level, she wanted desperately to believe that he was right, that she needn't continue with these horrible, enervating treatments, that there was another, better way.

"Well, here's where Sam and I take off," he said. He scribbled his home phone number on the back of his business card. "Call me, Robin, if you need anything. Anything at all."

"I may very well do that," she said, but she knew that if she ever did call him it would be as a desperate gamble. The Last Resort.

Robin had had this particular roll of pictures in her desk drawer for months before she got around to developing it. That's the way she was. She could never balance her checkbook for more than fourteen days at a time, forgot appointments, and generally had not yet mastered some of the rudiments of "grown-up" behavior. Nor did she really intend to.

She paid for the pictures, and glanced curiously at the crisp pack of photos as she strolled uptown on Park Avenue.

Mark's words were reverberating in her mind. Her head ached perpetually, she had no energy, and little verve for life. She looked a wreck and felt it too. She had had enough. How long had it been? She could hardly remember. And what good did it do? Imagine if the disease came back anyway! Then this year of suffering would have been for nothing. She would have been better off to have spent the year feeling well. It certainly did some good . . . but on the other hand, if it was true what Mark said, and it destroyed your immune system? No one had told her that. Could it be that Leslie and Dr. Vogel were hiding this from her? Or maybe they themselves didn't know. She was sorry she had missed that health convention. But probably it would have turned out to be an assortment of sorry freaks, more comical than serious, with their Moonie-faces enraptured with the latest fad in self-improvement. Anyway, she hated sprouts of every variety and carrot juice turned her off.

It was just so damn confusing.

She was flipping through the thirty-six pictures nonchalantly as she walked, Barney laughing with his tail beside her. She was almost at the entrance to her house when she reached the last picture in the roll. The pictures started out in her apartment—goofy shots of her roommate and her boyfriend. They switched from there to pictures of the skyline taken from the Staten Island ferry when her little niece and nephew were in for a visit. The last shots on the roll were from her Fire Island vacation.

And the last picture stopped her in her track and made her gasp audibly. For it was taken on *the very day* she had "rediscovered" her tumor. And there she was, squinting into the sun, smiling in an open, carefree way. And worst of all, she was in that little lemon-colored bikini, which pushed her small breasts forward and outward enticingly. Peter had the Italian penchant for big-busted women and it was he, in fact, who had bought her that particular outfit for the trip. What there was of it. And she looked good, good in a way she would never look again.

After her operation she had turned down another chance to go to Fire Island, with many excuses and assurances that it was *not* because of her lack of a breast. In fact, at the end of the season she had gone swimming at Jones Beach with her roommate, and they had had a lot of fun—forced jollity, she now thought—over whether or not Robin's falsie would float her to the surface, turn her over on her side, or drag her under with its weight. It did none of these, and in fact, the one-strap, over-the-shoulder bathing suit she had found in the "mastectomee" boutique was quite attractive. If you found such things attractive.

Looking at this picture of her self now, not only two-breasted but so clearly healthy, happy, and carefree, made her incredibly sad. Before and after. She could suddenly see the dimensions of what she had lost. But there she was, with the sword of Damocles about to fall and lop off part of her anatomy and she was as stupid, happy, and carefree as a clam.

Tears started to flow, and then became an uncontrollable flood. She tore into the building, not even hearing the hello of Tom the doorman, whom she had greeted for ten years, or the touch of Paulie, the forty-year-old cerebral palsy victim who reached out to console her in the elevator.

Robin continued the treatment, but still it was wearing her down. In the first part of each month she would go every day to Vogel's office to receive her injections. During that time she would also take her Cytoxan pills. At first the effects were not all that terrible, an upset stomach now and then, but after a while she began to notice hair on her pillow. She had always been proud of her auburn-colored hair, and now she was going to be as bald as a billiard ball.

Vogel was concerned about the hair loss, but calmed her.

"I told you you may experience some hair thinning," he said a bit defensively.

"You call this thinning?" Robin almost screamed. "You can see my scalp right through. How the hell am I supposed to perform like this? God, I'm really a wreck," she said, and the depth of her unhappiness moved him.

"Just hang in, Robin," he said. "It's doing good, I'm sure it's doing good. And the hair will grow back as soon as you finish the therapy. You'll forget you ever had this problem."

So she hung in, week by week. She refused to wear a kerchief, as so many chemotherapy patients did: it was a matter of stubborn pride with her. Let the world know, I don't give a damn.

When she came down with a cold she showed up at Vogel's office in panic. "I think this chemotherapy is doing me in, Dr. Vogel," she complained. "It's destroying my white blood cells and I'm getting infections right and left."

Vogel was more concerned about this: a greater risk of infection could indeed be a consequence of chemotherapy, especially intensive treatment. But when he checked Robin's blood tests he found that her white blood cells were remaining quite normal throughout the treatment.

"I'm afraid of the long-term effects of this stuff. I think I've sacrificed my good health. I'll never be the same."

"Don't be silly, Robin," Vogel answered. "I'm telling you, you're going to be your chipper old self once you get off the drug. There are no sophisticated studies that show any long-term ill effects from this type of chemotherapy. You know, our object is not to get anybody sick. We want you to be able to *work*, to go about your business. Otherwise, it's not really a successful adjuvant therapy. Are you working?"

"Are you kidding?" she asked. "The job market is terrible."

One time when she came in she announced to Vogel that she wanted to get pregnant, to have a child.

He frowned. This was a problem he did not often encounter. Breast cancer was a disease that mainly affected women over thirty-five, past their childbearing years. But Robin seemed serious.

"You're not married, are you?" he asked.

"What the hell does that have to do with it?" she shot back. "I'm talking medicine, doctor, not morality."

He smiled. "I'm just concerned about you." He reflected that in all the time she had been coming to him he had never received a call from her family. He had spoken to the boyfriend once and found him pleasant enough, but Robin's sudden interest in a baby seemed to him to be a rather desperate psychological attempt to affirm life in the face of so much death.

"Is there any problem with my having a baby?" she asked.

"Well, I'm not aware of any studies—"

"I don't care about studies," she said. "Just tell me, is it dangerous?"

"Yes, it's dangerous," he said. "Certainly it's *impossible* while you're still on the medication."

"And if I still decided to?"

"The baby might come out malformed, Robin. And you yourself might not be able to hold up to the strain. Have you ever had a baby?"

She shook her head.

"Please, just forget about it for now. There'll be plenty of time to think about it when you're done with chemotherapy. And that won't be long now."

"That's easy for you to say, Dr. Vogel," she murmured. "But what about *after* the chemotherapy?"

"You'd have to wait awhile," he said, "for the drugs to clear from your system. That might take several months. After that, well, you're entering an unknown region. As I *tried* to say, I know of no studies that show possible effects on the children of chemotherapy patients. In your case, I doubt if we're dealing with doses high enough to make a difference—after you've discontinued treatment for a while. But there are so many different, complex problems involved here.

"For one thing, you would have to have chromosome analysis of the amniotic fluid to see if there was any problem before birth."

"You mean, I might have to have an abortion? I'm not going to have an abortion. I don't believe in them."

"Okay, Robin, do what you like. I'm not telling you to have an abortion—" He sighed. "Robin, please don't put me in this bind. I'm just trying to do the best for you that I can. You'll have to make your own decisions, though."

Finally, one night in late autumn Robin came into the office in her warm-up suit. She had been exercising in the park, and had then come down 96th Street, stopping off for her appointment at the chemotherapist on her way home.

"You're looking hale and hearty," said Vogel, as he prepared to give her her injection. He had never treated a patient in a warm-up suit before, and the whole idea of it tickled him. To him she was an archtypical bohemian.

"You think so?" she asked. "I feel like death warmed over. I go through hell every month, then spend weeks trying to recover from that, until it starts again. I'm telling you, this is bad stuff."

She stared at the picture above the couch as the needle went in. It was a familiar Norman Rockwell "middle America" scene: a boy with his pants down, studying the doctor's diplomas, while the doctor himself got ready to plunge in a giant hypo. Yuk yuk yuk. Very funny. I wonder how cute Norman Rockwell would have found cytotoxic chemotherapy?

Robin could feel the drugs going into her vein. Every day that week and the week before she had come to this place, and let them inject her like this. She felt terrible, despite the warm-up suit and the image she tried to project. Actually, she hadn't been jogging at all—just walking and trying to move her arms and legs to get some circulation going. She had this terrible tiredness and queasiness she had never yet succeeded in describing to anyone.

It felt like she had been pummeled by muggers. Everything ached. Her bones ached, and each part of her body seemed to rebel against the other. And yet, amazingly, on the tests, at least, she was not really sick. It didn't show up in Dr. Vogel's "objective" measurements. Did that make her a hypochondriac? She could tell by the way he looked at her that he discounted everything she said. I wonder how brave he would be if he was getting the shots instead of giving them! Mr. Cool. Why the hell did I ever let them talk me into this? She couldn't remember the reasons and when she finally did, she felt embarrassed by them. If I had know what I was getting into . . .

"Well, that's done," said Vogel, picking up her folder and getting ready to move on to the next patient. "See you next week? No, you're off next week?"

"You're right," she said. "It's done."

Something in her voice unsettled him. He had seen this before. "What do you mean, Robin? What's bothering you?"

"I'm done, Dr. Vogel. Finished. I can't take this anymore."

Vogel sat down again and sighed deeply. He knew that the problem was largely psychological. A woman undergoes an operation with its brutal physical and emotional scars and the next thing she knows they're throwing chemotherapy at her. Often she agrees to it because she is in a scared and weakened condition. But after some months she begins to recover from the scars, and the operation becomes a memory. She wants to put it all behind her. But the chemotherapy is a reminder of her condition—because of it she is still a cancer patient. Putting medications into her veins is a distressful reminder of her status as a victim. And so, when patients reject adjuvant chemotherapy it is rarely because the drugs themselves are intolerable. It is the situation that has become intolerable. He knew that, but how could he convey that to Robin, who was so headstrong and determined.

"Don't quit now on me, Robin," he said finally. "You'll be off for a few weeks. . . ."

"Off for a few weeks, then on for a few weeks. How long can I go on like this? How long have we been doing this? I can't stand it."

"Just finish the course," he said. "It's really in your best interest."

"Sorry, Dr. Vogel. I can't do it. I know I'm going to regret this if something happens, but, well . . ."

Just then Vogel started laughing uproariously. It was a sound rarely heard in his offices. Robin was confused.

Vogel shook his head. "This is funny, really funny. The nurse left me a note, but I didn't see it." He had his hand in her record. "This is it," he said. "This is it."

"What do you mean?" She was half laughing herself—it was catching—but half angry. Often these jokes turned out to be at her expense.

"You are finished," Vogel said. "You just completed your last monthly cycle of treatments. You're free. I don't want to ever see you again, you understand?"

It took a moment for Robin to grasp the significance of this: somehow her own internal clock had measured off the weeks, injection by injection, and sounded the alarm on the very day the treatments were supposed to end. Neither she nor the doctor had kept track, but it was over all the same.

Unable to restrain herself, she leaped up and threw her arms around the doctor's neck and gave him a kiss on his mustache. He blushed, not used to such demonstrations of affection. Robin paid part of her bill (she was still in debt to both Vogel and Strong, but both had deferred payment until she found a steady job), and sauntered out of the office. A thick, romantic darkness had descended over the city. She would be meeting Peter for dinner—now they would really have something to celebrate. She jumped up into the air and—effortlessly it seemed—ran the rest of the way home.

Dr. Strong

For Strong it was another one of those gray, wet Brooklyn afternoons.

Just a few weeks before he and his son David had driven up the Taconic State Parkway to look at the changing leaves. They had stopped off in Dutchess County to pick apples, but the apple crop had been a wipe-out that year, and there was almost no fruit on the trees. The grizzled caretaker of the orchards came out of the barn and gave them a broken pole with a wire claw at the end. He refused to take any money from them, since the orchards were officially closed. With that claw they managed to gather a few pathetic-looking apples, a meager bag that could probably be made into a pie if they could convince David's mother to bake one. Yet, strangely, they had more fun being alone together in this way than on other trips in which the orchards were crowded with raucous families, their bushel bags stuffed to the brim with healthy specimens.

Now, once again, the leaves of Prospect Park were dull brown and the chill of the oncoming winter was in the air. He had spent the afternoon seeing patients. Mrs. Gipe had come by: she had finished her chemotherapy and was on her way to South America to do some missionary work for the Witnesses. Her recovery had been truly remarkable. Night had come on faster than it had any right to, and soon it would be time to fight the traffic back to Manhattan. Just then the outside doorbell rang. Strong's mind wandered back to that evening, almost a year before, when the outside bell had rung under similar circumstances. He wondered whatever had happened to Jill Highland, the beautiful young woman with inflammatory CA. He had recently read an article in one of the medical journals about a new approach to that problem. It wasn't a cure, but it did offer some new ideas. He hoped that her physician—if she had one—had read the article as well.

"Dr. Strong," asked his nurse, Susan, over the intercom, "could you see one more? She says it's important."

Strong sighed: it had been a long day. But there were sometimes emergencies in breast surgery and besides, if the woman bothered to come out on a night like this it must be important, to her at least.

"Dr. Strong," said the woman, "I got your name from my union, the Amalgamated Clothing and Textile Workers." She was an attractive lady, perched somewhere between youth and middle age.

Her name was Viola Martinelli* and she came bearing a printed form from the union. It was a familiar "second opinion" request. Strong did quite a few of these for corporations or unions, which found that they could often save money by ruling out unnecessary surgery in this way.

On the top the form bore the name of the primary physician, a general surgeon unknown to Strong. His diagnosis was "breast tumor" and the recommended procedure was a biopsy.

"I don't know where this problem came from," said Mrs. Martinelli. "The next thing I know they're sending me in for surgery." Her eyes pleaded with him.

"Let's take a look," said Strong, leading her into the examining room. She took off her blouse and brassiere and lay back on the table. Strong felt over the affected breast, his fingers quickly honing in on the suspicious area.

"Is this it?"

Mrs. Martinelli nodded.

"Did the other doctor take a mammogram?" he asked.

*Name changed.

"No, nothing."

"Did he stick a needle in this?"

"He didn't," said Mrs. Martinelli. "He just said I had to have surgery, a biopsy, to have it out. But I'm afraid of operations," she added, as if Strong didn't know. "I'm afraid they're going to take off my breast," she whispered.

"Did you sign any kind of release?" he asked.

The woman hesitated. "I was so upset I don't know what I signed."

"Okay, calm down, Mrs. Martinelli. I'm going to aspirate this. You'll hardly feel a thing, and then we'll have a much better idea of what's going on."

When Strong had calmed her sufficiently he took a syringe and slipped it into the lump. Mrs. Martinelli winced and bit her lip. He then drew out some fluid from the breast. It was straw-colored.

A few minutes later he felt the breast again. He was not surprised to find that the lump was gone.

"Do you remember where the 'tumor' was?" he asked, unable to keep the triumph out of his voice.

She nodded, and Strong guided her hand to where the lump had been. The look of joy and gratitude on her face made all the aggravation of his job worthwhile.

"Where is it?" she asked. "It's . . . gone."

"Yes, that's because you didn't have a tumor at all," said Strong. "What you had was a cyst, a little fluid-filled sac. We'll have to check you every six weeks for a while. If it recurs three times then we'll have to operate to remove it. But the chances are you'll be fine now."

Strong completed the union form: second opinion, mammary cyst. Aspirated. No surgery indicated at this time. He then gave Mrs. Martinelli some literature on the Breast Health Program, including the *Bulletin*. It was a nice ending to a long day.

A week later he got a telephone call from Katherine Sweeney, an official of the Amalgamated union, ACTWU.

"I just got the second opinion form you sent in on Mrs. Viola Martinelli," said Sweeney.

"Anything wrong?" asked Strong.

"Quite the contrary," the union official said. "We've noticed that a high percentage of your second opinions come back recommending against surgery. In this case, for instance, there really was no basis for recommending a biopsy, was there?"

"None whatsoever," said Strong. "The first thing the doctor should have done was to make sure he was not dealing with a simple cyst."

"Mrs. Martinelli was so impressed," Sweeney said, laughing, "that she made a special trip in here to show me the literature on the Breast Health Program."

"That's great," said Strong.

"We're very impressed as well. We've got seven thousand female workers in the New York City area and we've been concerned for some time that they're not receiving adequate breast care. And so, to get to the actual purpose of my call, we were wondering if you could come in and discuss this with us."

"I'd love to," said Strong. He was excited: perhaps this was the break he had been looking for. The corporations, by and large, had been unresponsive to his pleas. Perhaps the unions would find the BHP a cost-effective way to provide their members with an important health benefit. Everyone could come out ahead: the unions would look good, the members would be provided for, and the BHP would grow.

"What exactly did you have in mind?" asked Strong.

"Well, that's what we'd like to explore with you," said Sweeney. "For starters, we would like to reprint parts of your *Bulletin* in our union newspaper."

"I'll check with my public affairs consultant, Dorothy Wayner," said Strong, "but I don't foresee any problems with that." Actually, he knew that Dorothy would be as overjoyed as he was.

"And we would like you to give lectures to our members right here in the union hall on Broadway. As often as once a week, if you think you could work that into your schedule."

Strong's schedule was packed solid, but to expand the BHP he could always find another hour somewhere.

"That sounds feasible," he answered.

"And then we'd like to discuss a larger collaboration. But for that we would like you to come in and meet with some of our top people. There might be interest, you see, in extending your program of total breast care to our members. This could offer you a very large population for the Breast Health Program. Also, Dr. Strong, we have good connections with other unions in the area. I'm sure they would be impressed by any successful plan you worked out with us."

"Well, let's take it step by step," said Strong.

"Step by step," repeated Sweeney. "And the first step is to get you talking to some of our officials, such as Ron Minikus and Claire Levitt. You know, I think we've got something very good here. And I guess we have Mrs. Martinelli to thank for whatever comes out of this."

"Yes, Mrs. Martinelli," said Strong, "and all the Mrs. Martinellis."

Mildred

Mildred was scheduled to receive what was called "sandwich therapy." This consisted of two weeks of chemotherapy, followed by five weeks of radiation, and then the rest of the year on chemo again. For the radiation treatments, she was schlepping into the city on the Command bus and then hoofing it, with her daughter, to Beth Israel, over on First Avenue and 16th Street. Carol had taken a leave of absence from Head Start just to help her mother through this crisis.

At first everything was strange and a bit frightening.

They followed the signs to the Stella and Charles Guttman radiotherapy department. After a few days, she and Carol learned to "follow the yellow brick road" (a painted yellow stripe) to the department. They also learned the little tricks, which series of stairs and corridors to take to avoid the crowded elevators.

The department was in the basement, and construction was underway. The corridors smelled of damp plaster, and an unpleasant and vaguely disturbing smell: it contrasted with the almost forced gaiety of the waiting room. Everything was bright yellow, orange, and white, including the framed prints on the wall. It was as if someone had read in a textbook on hospital interior decorating that these particular colors were cheerful,

and then interpreted this quite literally, with a vengeance.
The patients here seemed somehow more eccentric than in Brooklyn. A man on a stretcher was wheeled by. He was dressed in a hospital gown, but on his head remained a jaunty beret. Carol pointed this out to Mildred, and they had a good laugh at this.

"Dear, you can go in here and change," said a young technician sweetly. She handed her a seersucker dressing gown. Mildred sat in the corridor and looked at the other patients. Many of them were worse off than her. There was an old lady, her nearly bald white head intersected with carefully diagrammed purple squares and rectangles. It was like something out of a sci-fi horror movie, Mil thought. She shuddered. Yet the old woman herself seemed quite cheerful, kibbitzing with the staff. Very pale people, deathly pale, with puffy orange eyes. Mildred felt almost guilty for being *well*, or relatively well. Deep inside she wondered if she would look like this after they got done with her. No, she couldn't think that! That way lies despair. She would have to think cheerful thoughts, to keep on laughing and making other people laugh.

"Please come in here, into room three," said the technician. She led her by the arm and Mildred was asked to lie down.

She was suddenly confronted with a monstrous machine—the Clinac 18. She had seen a diagram of a machine, on the wall of the corridor. But she had paid it little attention, no more than to the neo-impressionist prints, or the various posted instructions to the staff.

Now she suddenly realized what they meant by radiation therapy and it was scary. A towering, curving piece of metal, painted a deceptively innocent cream color, with a computer TV screen above her ready to record some kind of score. Outside the room she had noticed a cheerful young man at a computer control console. He probably operated the monster.

"It's . . . big" was all she could muster. She had thought this would be a joke. People had told her radiation was simple, that you didn't feel anything at all. But she had a sudden impulse to flee: what the hell was she doing here anyway? Hadn't the operation been enough? What more did they want? They got their pound of flesh!

"Yes, we're quite proud of it," said the aide. "We have three high energy units here. Two of them are cobalt. This is the linear accelerator. It's made by Varian. You're lucky that you came here, Miss Rosenbloom. We get patients from all over the world."

"Lucky, lucky me. I can see that," said Mildred, with a touch of irony that flew over the girl's head.

"This machine cost over a million dollars. It can deliver a beam of either electrons or high-energy photons."

"Wonderful," said Milly. "And what do I get?"

"You get the electrons, dear. The photons would penetrate too deep. We don't need to treat your lungs or your liver. Are you ready?"

The aide turned Milly toward the wall, and then hurried out of the room. Milly studied the wall-sized mural of trees, mountains, streams. Cheerful and woodsy. She felt a light sweat on her face as she heard the hum of the silent, lethal beam cutting into her. But she felt nothing.

They gave her a card, like an old-fashioned report card.

Beth Israel Medical Center
You are requested to
Return to the Clinic . . .

And so every working day, for five long weeks, she came back to Beth Israel for radiotherapy to her sternum, neck, and chest wall, until it became almost second nature to her. Each day they entered the date of her next appointment. She tried to read, bringing her Danielle Steel or Judith Krantz with her, but she just stared at the page, reading the same sentence over and over again. She brought her knitting, but that too was impossible. Her mind was elsewhere and wouldn't let her relax. Once, while waiting, she had found Beth Israel's equivalent of a chapel—the Silberman Meditation Room. She went in and sat down, alone.

It was hushed, quiet. What does one do in a Meditation Room, she wondered. Meditate. She had never meditated in her life, at least not consciously. Should she pray? But for what? She knew she was so much better off than most. She saw the incredible misery around her, but she didn't like to take consolation from other people's unhappiness; such thinking had always struck her as barbaric. Mildred knew that as long as she had her family, and especially her loving Phil, nothing could be so terrible. All would be for the best.

Moments passed. Suddenly a smile broke out on her face. Hey, she thought, I meditated! How do you like that?

Finally, what made the experience tolerable was that it *was* an experience. She and Carol made each trip into an adventure, the way they used to do when Carol was a teenager and they would go into the city on a shopping spree.

"What the hell, let's have fun," was Mildred's attitude.

They talked to the other patients, consoled them, listened to their problems. And they discovered some incredible people. There was a lawyer, so young and beautiful, who was taking courses of radiation on her lunch break from the courts.

"Can you believe that gal?" Carol said, as the woman went in to lie down under the big machine.

"God, I was so scared when I first went in there. But, like anything else, I guess you can get used to it."

"You're terrific, Ma," said Carol. She wondered, if it was her, whether *she* would be able to go through with this ordeal.

One day, on the No. 2 Command bus, she ran into an old friend, Gert.

"Where have you been, Mil? Haven't seen you around. How are you feeling?"

"Better," said Mildred, who assumed that all her friends knew about her mastectomy. Word of this sort of thing spread quickly in neighborhoods like Canarsie.

"Better than what?" asked Gert.

"Better than I did before," said Mildred.

"Say, listen," said Gert, remembering something and forgetting to ask the next obvious question. "Do you want to hear a joke? It's a good dirty one," she added, *sotto voce*. The lower the voice, the dirtier the joke.

"There's nothing I like more than a good dirty joke," said Mildred, laughing.

The three women huddled together in the back of the creeping express bus, giggling like pre-teens.

"A woman goes to her doctor, whose name happens to be Dr. Rosen, and says, 'Doc, I want you to make my tits grow bigger.'"

"I heard this one," said Carol, "but that's okay. Tell it again. I want to hear it again."

Gert seemed a bit perturbed, but continued, addressing herself to Mildred.

"She wanted to make her tits grow, see. And so Dr. Rosen says, 'Every day I want you to touch your hands to your shoulders, then up in the air, like this.'" She demonstrated a basic arm-lifting exercise. "'And repeat what I tell you, in rhythm. "Mary had a little lamb, whose fleece was white as snow. And if I do this every day, I'm sure my tits will grow." Well, she's going along doing this until one day she's in a hurry, see, and so she forgets to do her exercise. She's on the train and she decides to do them there. So very quietly, she raises her hands up and down—" Gert demonstrates. "—and says 'Mary had a little lamb whose fleece was white as snow and if I do this every day I'm sure my tits will grow.' She says it quietly, but a man sitting next to her hears her and says excitedly, 'Hey, you must go to Dr. Rosen.'

"The woman says, 'How do you know?' and so the man, the man—" Gert is gasping for breath and can hardly deliver the punchline. She slides out of her seat and stands in the aisle to demonstrate. "The man rotates his hips and says, 'Hickory, dickory, dock . . .'"

They all laugh hysterically. "Get it? Hickory, dickory, *dock* . . . pretty funny, huh?"

Mildred smiled: she just couldn't resist. "Gert," she said nonchalantly, "if I say that nursery rhyme do you think my tit will grow back?"

Gert's laughter froze. "Oh my God, Mil. Do you mean . . . that's what was wrong? Gee, I'm sorry, I'm really sorry," and she disappeared behind the high seat for the rest of the trip. Mildred winked at Carol and they had a good laugh of their own.

It was just when Mildred was getting comfortable with the radiation therapy, almost (but not quite) enjoying her daily excursions into the city, that it all came tumbling down.

One day, while she was dressing for her appointment, she noticed that she was sunburned on her shoulder—which was peculiar because it was already autumn and she hadn't even been out in the sun all summer. She touched the red area and realized that it covered a large area, precisely where the radiation beam was aimed.

When she went into the radiation clinic that day she showed the burned area to Dr. Myron Nobler, her radiologist and chairperson of the department of radiotherapy. Dr. Strong also came to look at the problem and to offer medical and moral support. Nobler and Strong studied it carefully, talking between themselves. Finally Nobler said, "As we told you when you began the treatment, Mildred, this type of radiation burn sometimes occurs. It's a transient condition, however."

"Does that mean it's going to get better?"

"It will get better, but I'm afraid that before it does it will get somewhat worse."

"Worse?" said Mildred. "It hurts like the dickens already, Dr. Nobler." She looked over to Strong in a silent appeal.

"It's temporary, Mildred," he said. "It might color the skin somewhat and perhaps thicken it a bit, but that's a small price to pay for the benefit it will give you."

"But what am I supposed to do now?" she asked plaintively.

"You'll have to apply a dressing to it each day. I'll show you how," said Strong. "But if it gets too bad, we can stop the treatment for a while. We'd rather not, because that might lessen the effect on the cancer cells."

And it did get worse. Now, instead of going uptown to Lord and Taylor or B. Altman's, she and Carol hurried home. Every bump on the bus was agony, as her blouse scraped against the red area. And just her luck, the weather turned unusually warm at this time. She sweated and chafed and suffered.

When she got home she could hardly make it up the three flights of stairs to her apartment. Carol helped her undress. She didn't want anything on her, but she couldn't walk around with nothing on—not with that terrible scar on her chest.

She put her feet up on the coffee table, knocking over the glass vase with the pink feathers sculpted into the shape of a flower bouquet.

"It's nothing, Ma," said Carol, but Mildred cried bitterly. "I never expected this, Carol, never. Strong warned me about this, but I guess I didn't believe him. I thought this was going to be a piece of cake. But now they're roasting me like a piece of meat." She laughed. Have to keep laughing. She hugged the big stuffed teddy bear she kept on the living room couch, and stared up at the water stain on the ceiling.

"Ma, do you want something to read?" said Carol. "Want *Love's Tender Fury?*"

"I'll just sit here. I'll be okay, doll. You can go home, go make dinner."

"Are you sure you'll be okay, Ma?" Carol asked.

Her face was so serious that Mildred had to laugh.

"I'll be okay," said Mildred. "Your father will be home from the luncheonette soon. He'll help me."

Philip worked part-time in a luncheonette since his retirement as a maintenance man for the Board of Education. They themselves had owned a luncheonette on Clarkson Avenue many years before, and he was happy to be back in the business, even if for a few hours.

When he came in, she was lying in the bedroom, suffering. She knew the bandage needed changing. She also knew she couldn't do that alone. The moment had come. They would have to confront this hurdle, she and Philip.

"How's my doll today?" he asked, kissing her. "Terrible weather, eh? Indian summer. I've been *schvitzing,* sweating, all day."

"Phil, I have to talk to you, sweetheart."

He sat down on the edge of the bed.

"I talked to the doctor about that tender area," she said. She had not exactly lied to him, but had not told him the full truth, either. Only that her chest and shoulder were "tender."

"What's up?" he said, sensing danger.

"He said . . . well, it's a burn from the radiation. It's quite normal, Phil. They say most people get it."

"But you've been so good these last few weeks."

"Well, I talked to some of the other patients. They say you get three good weeks at the start, three, three and a half weeks in which you don't feel any pain. Then—zingo! That's what's happening to me."

"Can I see the burn?" he asked slowly.

"Are you sure you want to? I mean, you're no *shtarker* when it comes to illness, Phil."

He laughed. "I promise not to pass out," he said. "I think I can stand the sight of you."

"Very funny," she said.

He encouraged her with his eyes, though, and she slowly removed her light gown, peeling it gingerly away from the wounded area.

"Oh my God," Phil said when he saw it. "What have they done to my baby?"

He wasn't looking at the bra with the prosthetic device where her breast had been, but at the ruby-red area—almost purple, it seemed—above it. He was speechless.

"Pretty bad, huh? Hurts like the dickens, too. I think if I'd known about this before I started the treatment . . ." She didn't finish the thought.

"God, I can't believe that. Why didn't you say something, Mil? And do you mean they gave you another treatment on *top* of that?"

"They have to, Phil. They have to try to get all the cancer 'bugs' while they still can. That's the whole point. They said they would stop, though, if it got really too bad."

"And *this* isn't too bad. I mean, that's going to *blister!*"

"It's blistering a little already. You can see over here. Jeez, Phil, I didn't think this would happen to *me*. I mean, I *tan*, I don't *burn*. I've never had a sunburn in my life."

"Maybe that's because you never sat under an accelerator before in your life," he said, and they both laughed. Her eyes glowed warmly: she could feel his love.

"I guess they know what they're doing. You know, you hear that this radiation therapy is so simple, but I see now that it's not," Mildred said.

"But, Phil, what I wanted to talk to you about is this—I'm going to need your help."

"Anything," he said in a low voice.

"I need you to dress the wound. The whole bit. The mastectomy, Phil." She paused, staring at him. "Can you do it?"

She was scared. As much as she knew he loved her, she dreaded a scene, a rejection, even after all these years. She knew how he felt about medicine and doctors, and until then she had made sure to change her bandages only when her husband wasn't around.

But he simply said, very naturally, "What's there to do? Wouldn't you do the same for me?"

Tears came to her eyes.

"They gave me something called Aquafor, it's a kind of Vaseline. You have to help me put that on the burn. Then we have to put another one of these xeroform pads on."

Together they removed the adhesive strips. She shut her eyes as the last strip came off and her breast—or rather the long straight scar where her breast had been—was exposed to view.

Phil stared at it for a long time, or what felt like a long time. This was the first time she had let him see it.

He didn't know what to say. He felt an incredible, almost tender, sadness: my poor Mil, my poor baby, what have they done to you? But he didn't want to say that. Because he also felt that it wasn't so terrible. She had survived the surgery. She would survive the radiation, and the chemotherapy, too, when they started to throw that at her. *They* would survive—together.

She opened her eyes.

He very gently began to apply the ointment. It hurt to have the wound touched, but it felt wonderful to feel his hands on her. Everything would be okay, she knew that now. The worst was over with. In a few weeks these burns would heal, her radiation would be over, and she would start to return to normal. His hands went over her in a circular motion, and she tried to relax a little bit.

When he was done, they lay in the darkened room for a while, side by side. There were mental scars, just like physical scars, and they both knew these would take time to heal.

They lay there silently, the two of them, listening to the noise of the traffic outside, together as they had been for forty-four years.

Finally, almost inaudibly, Phil whispered:

"We're going to make it."

Ten Years of Change:
An Interview with Dr. Leslie E. Strong

Q   In the 10 years that have passed since this book was first written many things have happened. But first tell us what most readers will want to know—what happened to the six women of *Stories of Hope and Healing* in the last decade?

A   Four of them are alive and well, with no sign of cancer. Tragically, two of them died—Robin Mack and Mildred Rosenbloom, each after a long and heroic battle against the disease. Robin survived a little over five years after diagnosis; Mildred about six years. Each, as the reader will remember, had cancers which had already metastasized (spread) when they first were diagnosed. Treating such cancers is still difficult, although today we have treatment options that were not available a decade ago.

Q   Probably the most dramatic change, from the public's point of view, is the growing incidence of breast cancer. In 1993, it was announced that at current rates, *one in eight* American women would develop the disease during her lifetime. Many of us had hardly gotten used to *one in nine*. About ten years ago the figure was one in twelve. It seems like a veritable epidemic. What's going on?

A   Breast cancer is increasing at about 3 percent per year, and we don't know why. In 1993, there were 182,000 new cases and 46,000 deaths from the disease. This is 32 and 18 percent, respectively, of cancer incidence and deaths among women. Breast cancer remains the most common form of cancer among women. This is not even counting the more localized *carcinomas in situ*, which would add an additional 25,000 cases per year.

Q   Is this a real increase, Dr. Strong, or are we simply seeing what is called a statistical artifact, created by the fact that today we have better and more aggressive early detection and screening programs?

A   Some of the increase is probably due to better screening programs detecting tumors before they become clinically apparent. But I believe there are other factors at work that are leading to a real increase in incidence. These may be environmental in nature—pollution, faulty diet, that sort of thing. If you look at Long Island, especially Nassau County, you find one of the highest incidence rates of breast cancer in the entire country. In that relatively affluent area, breast cancer is rising, compared to the five borough area of New York. It is distressing that we do not know why that is. Concerned women and their supporters in Congress are fighting to have a special Breast Cancer Task Force set up to find out why that is.

Q   So clearly new ideas are needed to deal with this epidemic. The Breast Health Program (BHP) of New York is one such concept. Could you reiterate for us the basic principle of this organization you founded?

A   Our basic concept was, and is, for women to have a physical breast examination and a diagnostic mammogram, with the correlation of the results of both procedures, in the same office visit. In this way, the patient gets all the results at the same time. The more common alternative is for the woman to go to her general practitioner, who then sends her to a radiologist, who does the mammogram, and then gives the results back to the primary care physician. He or she then has to interpret the findings and see whether or not to refer the patient to a general surgeon, and so forth. In this way, the patient may never get to see the right person in the first place.

Q   Put that way, it certainly sounds complicated. But what are the advantages of doing it the BHP way?

A   The BHP way involves less running around for the patient, less wear and tear. It is also more cost effective, because the patient only has to see *one* physician, who is a specialist, and everything needed is done at one time in one place. To reiterate: in one office visit, the woman gets a breast exam, a mammogram, and the results of both. In the other, more common way, she has to have at least three office visits.

Q   How would you compare the cost?

A   The BHP way is much less expensive—at least 50 percent less expensive than going for the three visits. Those three visits will probably cost the woman about $500. A BHP diagnostic visit is often around $250. Multiply that savings by the millions of breast exams that are given and you can see that the cost savings to society if it adopted our program would be enormous. At least, tens of millions of dollars in savings each year. Equally as important, women would probably get *earlier diagnosis* and *better treatment.*
That is because the patient would be seen from the start by a breast surgeon, who specializes in these kinds of cases, and by a radiologist, who only reads mammograms and therefore has the expertise in doing this procedure with certified, state-of-the-art mammography equipment. All of these factors are presently very cost effective.

Q   Yet the vast majority of doctors not only don't use that approach but some in fact look down upon it. How can you explain that odd situation?

A   Their criticism is that we are taking work away from radiologists, and that we are acting in a way that leads to the ordering of unnecessary mammograms, doing unnecessary procedures. The critics of our integrated approach are looking at the way that a person could abuse such an approach rather than the benefit of such an approach.

Q   Are there people who do abuse the system in this way?

A   Of course there are. The system is being abused in many ways: I get mammograms sent to this office from centers that are not approved, that are not accredited, where the quality of the mammography is very poor, and the reports are so poorly written that they do not correlate with the x-rays that I am looking at. It's very hard to explain that to the patients who bring these x-rays to me.

Q But aren't the indications for a mammogram fairly standard? The American Cancer Society (ACS) has issued certain widely disseminated criteria: a baseline exam between 35 and 40; a mammogram every two years between 40 and 50; and then one every year after 50....

A Right. But isn't it amazing that the majority of physicians today do *not* follow the procedures set forth by the ACS on mammography. Sadly, women have come to our office with lumps of which their doctor has been aware. But he or she said, "It can be watched," or "It's just fibrous tissue." And incredibly, some of these women have tumors that are indeed cancerous! *Lives* are being lost in this way and more often than we'd like to see. I've had patients come to this office with such stories.

Q Does this happen with pregnant women?

A Yes. The physician in such cases may not refer the patient to a breast surgeon, assuming that the growth is part of lactation, her pregnancy, or that a cyst is part of the pregnancy. Only after the pregnancy do they find out that the growth is still present and indeed requires a breast surgeon's evaluation. Over the years, I have had such patients referred to me, especially pregnant women, I'm sad to say.

Q If they had come to you first, what would have happened?

A They would have had an immediate biopsy. Pregnancy does not interfere with doing a biopsy, since it can be performed under local anesthesia, on an ambulatory, out-patient basis. They can be treated for cancer at that time, rather than to wait nine months, as pregnancy often has very deleterious effects upon breast cancer.

Q Are you talking about so-called "hormone-dependent" cancers?

A Correct. The growth of some cancers is very sensitive to an increase in hormones such as estrogen. That's why pregnancy is a very important time to diagnosis any breast abnormality. Through the BHP we have tried to spread the word that there are various myth about breast cancer and pregnancy—that breast lumps should be ignored in pregnancy and among nursing women. That's the first myth. The second myth is that breast cancer has a terrible prognosis if it is diagnosed during pregnancy. But breast cancer only has a terrible prognosis if you leave the tumor for nine months in a hormone-rich environment, which happen to be where the statistics are coming from. Many people still attribute it to cyst formation and do not undertake further diagnostic efforts.

Q But can one safely take a mammogram during pregnancy?

A No, you cannot. But if she feels a lump, the woman should see a breast surgeon, a specialist, to confirm or corroborate these findings. Most of the time, unfortunately, that does not happen.

Q So how can you diagnose breast cancer during pregnancy?

A The only way is to do a biopsy. With today's technology, that biopsy carries a negligible risk to the fetus. And it can be life-saving for the mother, especially with the new treatments that are becoming available.

Q What are some of the new chemical and hormonal treatments?

A Today we use tamoxifen (Nolvadex®), which is a kind of anti-estrogen. It is now used in both node-negative patients (whose lymph nodes show no sign of cancer) and node-positive patients, both pre-menopausally and post-menopausally. We believe that tamoxifen is important in delaying tumor recurrence and it is also very beneficial in combination with chemotherapy.

We have definite evidence that, in the post-menopausal woman, tamoxifen is the drug of choice, and it certainly gives added survival to such women. And in the pre-menopausal woman, the use of tamoxifen and chemotherapy for node-positive patients, certainly has added to the disease-free interval and has lessened recurrence. Depending on how one interprets the statistics, one could actually say there has been an increase in overall survival in certain stages of breast cancer.

We have advanced in the use of another drug, called taxol, which is derived from the Pacific Yew tree. This is a very new experimental agent for advanced breast cancer.

In the field of chemotherapy, I could summarize it by saying we have new agents, we have a greater ability to treat patients. Whereas before we only treated node-positive patients, today node-negative patients are also being treated to prevent recurrence and to increase survival. We have better chemotherapeutic regimens for these patients.

Q Is breast self-examination (BSE) the best way to find a tumor early?

A Routine BSE is important. The whole point of modern treatment is to get early diagnosis, before the cancer has spread. That way, the tumor can be removed before it spreads to other organs. Treatment of what is called disseminated cancer is much more problematic. That is why it is important to teach women how to examine their own breasts on a monthly basis for incipient growths. At the BHP we distribute a handy shower card that reminds women to perform BSE while they are showering or bathing.

BSE alone is not enough, however. We urge women to follow the American Cancer Society's recommendations on mammography as well. These urge women to have a baseline mammogram (a radiological picture of the breast) some time between the ages of 35 and 40, another mammogram once every two years between the ages of 40 and 50; and then a mammogram every year after the age of 50.

Q Isn't there a danger from all that radiation?

A In the last 10 to 15 years, mammograms have become much safer. Today, in expert hands, at a qualified center, they deliver a fraction of a rad of radiation. There is no evidence that that little amount of radiation can do harm to the vast majority of women.

Plus, we are seeing the emergence of machines that deliver even smaller—infinitesimal—amounts. These are called ultra-high-frequency mammography machines. They utilize a regular household current and are so safe they no longer require lead-lined rooms.

Q   So women should go to their doctor for mammograms...

A   Time out! I don't mean to insult any general practitioners or gynecologists, but I think it is very important that a woman should see a breast *specialist* for her breast examination. After all, there are heart specialists, kidney specialists, ear/nose/throat specialists and today breast specialists.

Q   What's involved in this specialization?

A   We at the Breast Health Program of New York believe in a multidisciplinary approach to the appropriate care of the breast. This means, first of all, to see a surgeon who specializes in that area; to have a thorough physical examination by someone who does constant breast exams; followed by a high-quality mammogram, which then can be immediately correlated with the physical findings.

Q   Is this what most women are getting today?

A   Sadly, no. In fact, only about 20 to 30 percent of women are getting regular mammograms—and that includes x-rays taken in malls and in mobile units.

Q   So you feel that there is much room for expanding the national mammography program. But wouldn't that be too expensive, especially in this era of medical cost-cutting?

A   That is a misconception. First of all, finding cancer early is hardly as expensive as trying to treat it in its disseminated phase. That can run into more than a hundred thousand dollars per patient—and even today is rarely very successful in terms of life extension. *Prevention, early diagnosis and early treatment are the most cost effective thing we can do in breast cancer management.*

Q But what about this question of cost? I understand that a check-up plus a mammogram will run about $500...

A That is, only if you separate your visits as stated previously, rather than consolidating your visit to one specialist. Here at the Breast Health Program of New York we follow a multidisciplinary approach. This means that we have state-of-the-art mammography on site. A skilled breast surgeon then correlates the results with the physical breast findings. A board-certified radiologist reads the mammograms, right then and there. This can be done for less than half the cost of the usual office visits, and saves the woman a lot of running around.

Q Dr. Strong, let's talk frankly. Isn't this exactly the approach that was criticized in a recent book on breast cancer. In fact, they have a special pull-out in a box that warns readers not to have a mammogram in the office of a surgeon who has a mammography machine on premises. Wouldn't that apply to you?

A Yes, and this is an ongoing struggle within the field. The criticism of a doctor for having his own mammography machine is like prohibiting a cardiologist from performing an electrocardiogram (EKG), or a pulmonary specialist from performing a chest x-ray. These are the specialist's tools, without which he cannot make a comprehensive diagnosis. There is also a legitimate concern that the surgeon him/herself is unqualified to read the x-ray. That is why here at the BHP we employ an expert radiologist to read the results. There is also a concern about unnecessary procedures when doctors own their own equipment. But, in fact, we know well the parameters for mammography—they are agreed upon by most experts. We are not doing routine mammograms on, say, 20-year-old women. We are only giving them when they are indicated by, for example, the ACS guidelines.

Q That can't be all there is to it!

A No, of course not. The real reason, I believe, is the fear among certain elements in the medical profession that combining examination and radiology in one location would infringe upon the radiologists. Perhaps. But I don't think that is a sufficient reason to put the women themselves to the considerable trouble and expense of multiple visits, running from one end of town to another. To me, if something is your specialty, you should have the appropriate equipment to do it. I'm not solely reading the x-rays. I also have a radiologist do that. But the criticism is that you're doing unnecessary x-rays for your own financial gain. That you're doing unnecessary procedures.

Q Would you describe some of the treatment advances that have been made since 1984?

A First of all, there is tamoxifen—Nolvadex®—a drug that is now used in both pre- and post-menopausal women. Tamoxifen delays tumor recurrences, led to a greater disease-free interval and increased overall survival in some stages of cancer. And is beneficial with chemotherapy, as well. In post-menopausal women, tamoxifen is the drug of choice.

Another exciting innovation of the last few years is taxol, a plant derived from the Pacific yew tree.

Q On another topic, we've heard alot about DCIS. What is it?

A DCIS stands for ductal carcinoma-in-situ. This is also called "stage 0" cancer. A carcinoma is the most common kind of cancer, while in-situ means that it is confined to the ducts of the breast. It means it has not infiltrated. These are sometimes called "precancerous," but that term is highly misleading term. Such cancers can be cured when treated at this stage, with a cure rate of 95 to 97 percent.

DCIS was rarely seen before mammography became more common. We now know a lot more about it. DCIS generally does not require a mastectomy. It can simply be treated with either a lumpectomy or a quadrantectomy, followed in some cases by radiation treatment, but definitely no axillary (under the arm) node dissection. This is a major advance in treating patients.

Q How often does DCIS progress to actual cancer?

A If it is left untreated, however, it can progress to infiltrating duct carcinoma over a period of years. The two more aggressive kinds of DCIS are the comedo and cribriform. These are treated with wide excision and radiation. The less aggressive kinds are the tubular and the solid. These are generally treated with lumpectomy.

Q How is DCIS found?

A It first usually shows up as microcalcifications of the breast, which are best diagnosed by routine mammography, routine breast exam, picking up a focus of microcalcifications in the breast. This is simply cured by removing the calcifications through a lumpectomy or, if it is more extensive, through a quadrant resection. As long as the remaining breast is free of microcalcifications that breast can then be treated with radiotherapy, or with observations, depending on whether it is more aggressive (the comido or cribriform type) as contrasted with the more benign (tubular or solid) type.

Q Why is DCIS becoming more common?

A Because of the more sophisticated mammography equipment that we have now we are seeing more of it. We are now able to find smaller foci of microcalcifications than we were ten years ago.

Q And what is LCIS?

A LCIS stands for lobular carcinoma-in-situ. This is generally a bilateral disease, i.e. is found in both breasts simultaneously. It is usually an incidental finding at the time of biopsy or at the time of a mammogram, when you find a focus of microcalcification. At that time you may also find incidental foci of LCIS. We now know that LCIS can be treated non-surgically. In the overwhelming number of cases these women do just as well as other women—just with regular mammograms. There is *no* increase in mortality by following LCIS in this way. This is in contrast to what is sometimes recommended, a bilateral prophylactic mastectomy, i.e. the "preventative" removal of both breasts. LCIS is simply a marker for increased risk. About 20 percent of the women who have this symptom go on to develop an infiltrating cancer over the next 20 to 30 years. That is why they have to be watched very carefully.

Q What other advances have been made in breast surgery?

A We now have proven that breast-preserving operations definitely cure the early stages of breast cancer. These have replaced modified radical mastectomies in such early stages. These were generally not available ten years ago. This was controversial a decade ago; now it is an established fact. We can use these breast preserving operations for DCIS and we can definitely use it also for Stage I Breast Cancer and early Stage II Breast Cancer. Stage I is a small tumor, under two centimeters in size, with no cancer in the lymph nodes, while early stage II consists of tumors two to three centimeters in size. We can operate now with minimal or no deformity.

Q All these new operations are expensive. Have there been any improvements in insurance coverage for breast cancer treatments?

A Yes. We now have complete insurance coverage for reconstructive surgery of the breast. Ten years ago, some insurance companies would not approve such operations. Breast reconstructive surgery is no longer considered just cosmetic, as it once was, and is approved by all insurance companies. It is considered part of the treatment of the cancer patient.

Q Has the method of reconstructing patients changed?

A It is far more sophisticated. We now have the use of what is called a TRAM flap, the trans-abdominal muscle flap. In this procedure, we actually move the abdominal musculature to the chest. We use the rectus abdominus muscle, which is the abdominal muscle, to fashion a breast. We do not in many cases have to use a breast prosthesis. The TRAM flap has revolutionized reconstructive surgery. It has avoided the use of prosthetics.

Q Does this adversely influence abdominal tone?

A If you use one rectus muscle, in what is called a unipedical flap, it does not injure the abdominal musculature, because you still have the opposite abdominal rectus muscle. If you use a bipedical flap, which is both muscles, then you obviously have a weakness to the abdominal musculature, because the muscle is not present. But we offset that with what we call a "tummy tuck" procedure, so that the abdomen is made flat and the patient has an excellent cosmetic result.

Q   What kind of breast prostheses are used?

A   We used to use a dual implant, made of saline and silicone. Because of the health problems with silicone, causing auto-immune illnesses, however, we are now basically using the saline implant for those patients who are not candidates for a TRAM flap. The saline is encased in a plastic which, as far as we know, is inert.

Q   On another topic, what sort of advances have been made in the prognosis of breast cancer?

A   For prognosis, we have a dozen tumor markers available today. Only a few of these were known ten years ago, such as Estrogen Receptors (ER) and Progesterone Receptors (PR). Some others were experimental, while yet others were in the realm of science fiction just a decade ago. Some of these are in general use now, while others are still for investigational use only. The approved solid tumor tests include the following:

1. DNA Index (DI): Abnormal DNA content that identifies an aggressive cancer and tells if there is a greater risk of early recurrences.

2. S-Phase Fraction (SPF): If there is a high percentage of what are called S-phase cells, this indicates a poorer prognosis.

3. Cycling Index (CI): If there is a high rate of cell proliferation this also indicates an aggressive tumor that has a greater risk of recurrence.

4. Proliferating Cell Nuclear Antigen (PCNA): This is another proliferation marker that is used in paraffin embedded tissue. A high rate of proliferation of cells shows that there is an aggressive tumor with a greater risk of recurrence.

5. *Estrogen Receptor (ER)*: ER positive tumors are more likely to respond to hormonal therapy.

6. *Progesterone Receptor (PR)*: These may detect false negative ER results in frozen tissue. This is better correlated with the outcome of endocrine therapy.

7. *Epidermal Growth Factor Receptor (EGFR)*: This helps to sort patients into favorable and unfavorable prognostic groups.

In addition, there are five investigational markers that are proving to be of great importance:

8. *Estrogen Regulated Protein (pS2)*: These may detect some false negative ER results in paraffin embedded tissue. If there are increased levels, these are associated with increased overall and disease-free survival.

9. *HER-2/neu Oncoprotein (H2n)*: An overexpression of this oncoprotein often predicts poor survival.

10. *Cathepsin D (Cath D)*: This is a lysosomal enzyme that indicates a shortened recurrence-free survival period.

11. *Multiple Drug Resistance Testing (MDR)*: Elevated levels of this protein often indicates resistance to chemotherapy.

12. *Tumor Suppressor Gene (p53)*: An overexpression of this protein is associated with a shortening of disease-free and overall survival times.

Both I and the medical oncologist now have more ways of following the patient, and predicting how she will do. The activity of the DNA of the tissue can now be analyzed. Is it diploid or aneuploid? Aneuploid is a worse prognosis than diploid. We now go through the S-Phase: how fast is the tumor's doubling time? We go through the NER-2/neu Oncoproteins. An overexpression of this oncoprotein also suggests a poor prognosis. We now have a way of analyzing breast cancer tissue better than we had before.

Q How does this affect the patient's outcome?

A For node negative patients, who have overexpression of oncogenes, for example, and have high S-phase and are aneuploid, even though they're node negative, they should be treated as though they are node positive. They would therefore most likely receive a course of chemotherapy and hormone therapy. This is in contrast to a node negative patient who is diploid, who has a low S-phase, who has no expression of the oncoprotein and no expression of Cathepsin—those patients would have less of a risk of recurrence, stage for stage. That is a major advance which adds another dimension to managing the breast cancer patient.

Q Which of these markers are currently routinely used in your practice?

A Estrogen, pS2, HER-2/neu, Cathepsin D, DNA analysis, S-Phase and the Cycling Index. We do a whole battery of tests on our patients. And these results are pretty much consistent with each other. When one is high, the others seem to fall into place. Ten years ago, we said that if a patient is estrogen receptor negative, she would not benefit from tamoxifen. Today, we believe that some patients who are estrogen receptor negative, but have poor scores on the other tests, can still benefit from this treatment.

Q Are there any other advances in early diagnosis?

A Yes, there is a relatively new technique called stereotactic needle biopsy, also known as the "thin needle aspiration." That is done on certain mammography machines, where you can see a tumor on a mammogram, which you may feel is completely benign (i.e., well-defined, round, smooth borders, less than one centimeter in size) and you would like to be sure if this is, in fact, benign or malignant. We now have a computer-guided machine which can place a needle directly into the tumor, aspirate the tissue, and tell the patient and the doctor if this is benign or malignant.

If it is benign, then that patient would not need to undergo operative intervention, but can just be followed by mammograms every six or eight months. Many benign "lesions" can be followed in this way, without the woman having to undergo a biopsy operation. This didn't exist ten years ago.

Q Is there any danger, if the growth turns out to be malignant, of tracking the cells with the needle?

A No. If it turns out to be malignant, the needle localization is then done and the tumor is removed. But there is no tracking of cancer cells through the needle track, because the patient is then followed within a week or so with a formal excisional biopsy. This is a very safe technique and is certainly of very great diagnostic as well as therapeutic value.

Q In treatment, isn't there a difference between disease-free interval and survival?

A Yes. Survival means how long a person actually lives; the disease-free interval is the time in which the person is free of a recurrence or metastasis. If we increase the disease-free interval that doesn't mean that we've actually increased the person's survival time. But at least if you can increase the disease-free interval, it demonstrates that we are on the right track towards an increase in patient survival. In the post-menopausal woman, that is very well established. In the pre-menopausal woman, it depends on what statistic you are reading. But there is a general feeling that the overall survival of the pre-menopausal woman is increased. It seems that for every 100 women who had a stage II breast cancer, according to a 1992 article in the *Lancet*, adjuvant therapy produced 12 additional ten-year survivors. The benefits were smaller for stage I disease, where the survival is thought to be 85 to 90 percent. In this group, adjuvant therapy produced 12 additional ten-year survivors for every 200 women treated. The concept in this *Lancet* article is that there seems to be an increase in survival through the use of chemotherapy and hormone therapy together.

In pre-menopausal women, however, you're correct: there doesn't seem to be that much statistical improvement, but in certain cases there are. The final answer is yet to be brought in, because we have so many new drugs that are being used right now to come up with those statistics.

Q   What about bone marrow transplantation?

A   That's the new method that has received a great deal of publicity. It involves giving people high doses of chemotherapy and/or radiation, and then following that with injections of fresh bone marrow from a healthy donor. It appears to be a "salvage" technique in some very advanced cases of cancer. But it also has a high mortality rate itself—about 25 to 30 percent of the people who get it do not survive the treatment. It is a very dangerous procedure and I am really not clear in my own mind of the indications for it. It is a last ditch effort. It is now being done in an increasing number of cases. Hopefully we will get some better results with it.

Q   The political aspects of breast cancer have been much in the news. How does the level of organization, professional and political, compare to a decade ago.

A   There is simply no comparison. Today, breast surgeons in my area have their own organization, The New York Metropolitan Breast Cancer Group, headquartered at Memorial Sloan-Kettering Cancer Center. This is a group mainly for breast surgeons. It shows that breast surgery is now a recognized subspecialty, where special training is appropriate after residency, to do work in breast cancer.

Q   Ten years ago, you seemed a bit beleaguered, in the sense that very few people were doing what you were. To be a breast surgery specialist *per se* was not widely recognized as a concept.

A   Correct. Today, however, it is better established. This awareness of the need for expertise in the treatment has been heightened by all the famous people who have had breast cancer. This has made our field more established. In oncology today we have experts in the chemotherapeutic treatment of breast cancer. These people treat only breast cancer patients. The whole field is moving towards specialization, at both the treatment and the follow-up level. This is a new development.